WHAT ARE YOU DYING FROM *THIS* WEEK?

HELP FOR HEALTH ANXIETY

Heather Shearer PhD

Copyright © 2018 Heather Shearer

All rights reserved.

ISBN: 9781792019883

Imprint: Independently published:

CONTENTS

WHAT ARE YOU DYING FROM THIS WEEK? help for health anxiety 1
    Introduction 1
    About the author 1

Chapter One: Health Anxiety 2
    What is anxiety? 2
    The history of health anxiety (and anxiety) 7
    What is health? 8
    Unhelpful assumptions 10
    So, what IS Health Anxiety? 11
    How do you know if you have health anxiety? 15
    When is health anxiety a cause for concern? 16
    Negative impacts of health anxiety 20

Chapter Two: Origins of Health Anxiety 24
    How Health Anxiety develops 24
    Parental modelling 24
    Being ill yourself 25
    Genetics and epigenetics 26
    Evolutionary biology – fight, flight or freeze 27
    Trauma 29

- Gut bacteria 29
- Risk perception 30
- Time orientation and health anxiety 30
- The media and the internet... 31
- Negatives of society.. 33

Chapter Three: What triggers health anxiety? 35
- Triggers 35
  - Someone being diagnosed or dying from a serious illness. 35
  - Medical checkups 36
  - Other stress in your life 36
  - Hormonal changes... 37
  - Change in diet.. 38
  - Alcohol (and drugs).. 39
  - Not being able to exercise 41
  - You DO have a health condition 42
  - Unhelpful Health Related Thoughts 43

Chapter Four: How health anxiety is maintained................................. 44
- Control... 44
- Catastrophising.. 45
- Checking 48
- Avoidance and safety behavior 52

- False stories (real but not true) 53
- Overthinking (over analyzing) 54
- Anxiety 55
- Chapter Five: Helpful things to do 57
  - Long Term Interventions 57
    - Counselling and Psychology 57
    - Medication 62
    - Exercise 67
    - Faith 69
    - Mindfulness (and Meditation) 71
    - Death Cafes 80
    - Volunteering 81
    - Talks and Podcasts 82
  - Crisis Intervention Techniques 83
    - Breathing and mindfulness techniques 83
    - What evidence do you have? 87
    - Tapping (Emotional Freedom Technique) 90
    - Anxiety Forums 92
    - Best Friend technique 94
    - What is the benefit of NOT finding out 95
    - Dumb ways to die 96

Conclusion 98
Stories of health anxiety 99
   THINGS I HAVE THOUGHT I WAS DYING FROM (AND THE REAL CAUSE)
.... 99
   a personal story of health anxiety 100
   REFERENCES 104

ACKNOWLEDGMENTS

Thank you very much to my best friend Dave, for always being able to make me come down to earth. Thank you too to Tara Brach, a wonderful wise teacher (who I have never met, but who inspires me every day). I only wish I had discovered your work years ago! I'd also like to acknowledge the BEST health anxiety resource out there: the Western Australian Centre for Clinical Interventions workbook, Helping Health Anxietyi. Finally, thanks to my great doctor, Dr G, who gave me the title for this book!

WHAT ARE YOU DYING FROM THIS WEEK? HELP FOR HEALTH ANXIETY

Introduction

If you are reading this, you are likely doing so because you or someone close to you has health anxiety. Health anxiety has always been the 'poor relation' of anxiety disorders, and at times, those of us with health anxiety are mocked by others, who call us hypochondriacs, or other cruel names. Even respected sources often do not include health anxiety in the list of anxiety disorders[i]. But health anxiety is a genuine, often debilitating anxiety disorder; which for many people, results in spending much of their lives feeling constantly stressed, worried and even having panic attacks.

This book will describe how health anxiety originates, how it is perpetuated, some ways to help with health anxiety and various stories from people with health anxiety. I'm also going to reference a lot from the best health anxiety resource that I have ever read; a series of modules created by the Western Australia Centre for Clinical Interventions called Helping Health Anxiety[ii]. The first part of the book discusses anxiety in general, and then goes on to discuss health anxiety.

About the author

Heather Shearer is an academic researcher and lecturer who works at Griffith University, Queensland Australia. She has a PhD in environmental science and behavioural psychology. She has diverse research interests, including the benefits of outdoor exercise on mental health, spatial information and data analysis, housing affordability, the tiny house movement, and long distance hiking and mental health.

As you can probably figure, I have health anxiety too!

CHAPTER ONE: HEALTH ANXIETY

What is anxiety?

Anxiety has now overtaken depression as the number one mental illness in the developed world, and it's increasing. One in 4 Australians report that they suffer from anxiety (1 in 3 women, and 1 in 5 men)[i].

A degree of anxiety is, of course, normal. Without any worries or fears, we'd be sociopaths, unable to feel any emotion at all. Humans are weak creatures, without fangs, claws or thick skin. We've evolved to naturally feel fear as a response to real or potential danger. Back when humans roamed the African savannah, we learned to fear things like a rustle in the bushes, the hiss of a snake, or a fire on the horizon. If we hadn't done so, we wouldn't have survived to pass on our genes to our children, and eventually to us.

Early humans, and sadly, many humans still today, live dangerous lives. If they are not constantly alert, they could get maimed or killed by wild animals, or worse, by other humans. Even today, many people live in constant fear of bombs, suicide bombers, gang violence or natural hazards. But most of us are lucky enough not to live in such conditions.

When we are genuinely threatened, we have a physiological response called fight-flight-freeze[ii]. If something threatens you, and you think you can defeat it, you can prepare do battle with whatever it is (fight); if you think it is too powerful, you can run away (take flight); or if it is utterly terrifying and you don't think even running away can help you, then you can freeze in terror and hope it doesn't see you (as do many wild animals). This response is hardwired, and it comes from the deepest, most ancient part of the brain, our reptilian brain (see box).

The Triune Brain[iii]

This theory is rather simplistic, and most neuroscientists nowadays don't really support this. Nonetheless, it's a good allegory for how we respond to stress. This differentiates the brain into three parts, in order of evolutionary age; the reptilian, mammalian and primate brain[iv].

The **reptilian** brain is the oldest, found even in ancient reptiles (hence the name), and controls vital functions such as heart rate, breathing and body temperature. It includes the brainstem and the cerebellum. The behaviour of the reptilian brain is unconscious and instinctive. The reptilian brain is the part of us that acts to avoid harm; it responds to threats, stress and environmental hazards. The reptilian brain is fundamentally concerned with the fear of danger; that something is going to go wrong, that we won't be able deal with what is going to happen, with the unknown. Ultimately, the fear is of loss, loss of our bodily selves.

The **mammalian** brain is found in mammals. It is often responsible for emotions and value judgments, as it stores memories of behaviours that either have pleasant or unpleasant outcomes. The mammalian brain contains the hippocampus, amygdala, and hypothalamus. This is important, as the amygdala is strongly connected with anxiety. The mammalian brain acts to enhance pleasure and to seek rewards. One way we deal with fear, is to seek reward, to make us feel better. The mammalian brain triggers our search for more comfort to deal with our fear; in ways that are temporary and bad for us, like drinking too much, taking drugs, shopping or gambling.

The **primate brain (or neocortex)** developed in primates and reached its (current) peak in the human brain. The cerebral hemispheres are thought to be responsible for language, abstract thought, imagination, and consciousness.

This part of the brain also has a great capacity to learn. The primate brain is concerned with attachment and connection to others. We use strategies to get attention and to seek approval and security. If we constantly want something *more* from people, ultimately no person or relationship can provide us with the security that we desperately seek.

Tara Brach likens the three brains to the Garden of Eden. The mammalian brain is seeking pleasure (eating the forbidden fruit), the reptilian brain is afraid of the consequences of eating the fruit, and the primate brain is scheming how to restore attachment to God by lying[v].

It is normal to be anxious about certain situations, such as giving a presentation to a group of strangers, getting married, going for a job interview, being in a stressful environment, such as high speed traffic, flying, going overseas for the first time, going on a first date, participating in a sporting event or meeting someone who you particularly admire.

However, some of us---due to past trauma, genetics or childhood adaptations to difficult circumstances---are overly sensitive to threats. Our fear button is constantly on, so that even the smallest things can make us anxious and fearful. So, if we are spending much or even most of our time worrying and stressing, and we cannot stop, then anxiety becomes a problem. In that case, anxiety interferes with our enjoyment of life, and can have negative impacts on our work and relationships and other parts of our life.

To some, the things that are of concern to anxiety suffers may seem trivial or unimportant, and situations are often viewed as much more negative or black and white than they are in reality. But it is very difficult for anxiety suffers to view some situations objectively. Moreover, there are different types of anxiety, and something that a person with health anxiety fears, say, having a terminal illness, may not be fearful at all to someone with social anxiety who is terrified of meeting strangers (and vice versa)[vi].

Anxiety is therefore not just one problem; it is a collection of related, but not identical, disorders. People can suffer from more than one type of anxiety, but generally, one type is dominant. Some of the commonest types of anxiety are detailed below[vii][viii]:

- **Agoraphobia.** An anxiety disorder where a person is afraid of leaving perceived safe environments, most commonly home. Busy public places are often terrifying, and sometimes people with agoraphobia become almost housebound for fear of triggering panic attacks.

- **Generalised Anxiety Disorder (GAD).** People with GAD tend to feel anxious or worried all the time, and these worries interfere with their normal day to day life. These worries are often over what non GAD anxious people think are very minor, such as household chores or running late.

- **Obsessive Compulsive Disorder (OCD).** Like health anxiety, OCD is often misunderstood, and those suffering from OCD often hide the condition for fear of being shamed or mocked. However, it is very debilitating, and the constant checking and/or compulsions can result in significant distress and difficulty with day to day living.

- **Panic Disorder.** Panic attacks can occur in any anxiety disorder and can be terrifying. Frequent, unexpected and disabling panic attacks are known as panic disorder. Panic attacks have overwhelming physical sensations, often akin to serious medical conditions. People with health anxiety may experience panic attacks.

- **Post-traumatic stress disorder** (PTSD). PTSD usually develops after a traumatic event, such as accidents, war experiences or assaults. It is very debilitating, and can result in intense fear, horror, nightmares, panic attacks, and helplessness. People with PTSD often have flashbacks to the traumatic event, are easily startled, and have sleeping difficulties.

- **Separation anxiety disorder.** This is more common in children under 12, but more rarely is found in older children and adults. It is characterized by fear and anxiety about being separated from an attachment figure (i.e. a parent or partner), or from home. It can result in physical symptoms such as nausea and nightmares.

- **Social phobia.** Social phobia is similar to GAD, and all people, to some extent, feel nervous in new social situations.

When it is considered a phobia however, is when it goes beyond mild fear into extreme anxiety about situations such as giving a speech, being watched at work or even social interaction.

- **Postpartum anxiety.** Unlike postpartum depression, postpartum anxiety is lesser known, but probably affects new mothers in about the same proportion. This is relatively common however, affecting approximately 15% of new (and pregnant) moms and 10% of dads. PPD and PPT should be taken seriously; in Australia, 20% of maternal deaths are from suicide. Like all forms of anxiety, sufferers can be stigmatized, particularly nowadays, with social media pressure to be 'perfect' mothers. More seriously, but more rarely, this can also manifest at postpartum psychosis.

- **Phobias.** It is normal and rational to be afraid of things that can kill you, such as venomous snakes or falling from heights, but when these fears are out of proportion to the actual object or event, then they are termed phobias. People with phobias (about almost anything) can suffer panic attacks and overwhelming physical sensations, even chest pain, sometimes when just thinking about the object of their phobia. Phobic people are normally aware that their fear is unwarranted and irrational, but are not able to control their automatic reactions.

A couple go to the doctor. After the husband's checkup, the doctor calls the wife into the office. "Your husband is suffering from extreme stress and anxiety, and if you don't do something, he'll surely die."

Extremely concerned, the wife asked the doctor what she could do. The doctor replied, "Every morning you must fix him a healthy breakfast. Then you must make him a nutritious lunch to take to work. While he's at work, you must keep the house is spick and span, so he doesn't come home to disorder. Never nag or discuss your problems with him, and always be cheerful. Every night, prepare and serve him a three course dinner, then give him a back massage, and make love for as long as he likes. If you do this for a year, he'll survive to a good old age."

On the way home, the husband asked the wife, what did the doctor say?

She said, "you are going to die"

The history of health anxiety (and anxiety)[ix]

In the era of the Ancient Greeks, anxiety was known as hysteria, which directly translated from the Greek, means 'unsettled uterus'. Throughout history, anxiety has always been prone to gender discrimination. Back then, it was thought to only affect women, and caused by the uterus wandering around the body, blocking off passages and affecting breathing. Another sexist interpretation then was that it was caused by 'female semen' which, due to lack of sexual intercourse, would collect in the body and turn to poison. The cure was, of course, sex (with a man only, of course).

By the middle ages, hysteria (still only affecting women) was not a good thing. Women with anxiety were often accused of being witches. If a woman was accused of being a witch or if they were too vocal about accusing other women of being witches, the 'treatment' for their anxiety included torture, execution or burning at the stake.

In the Victorian era, women were less likely to be considered witches (thankfully), and instead, were just treated as batty. If a woman had a lot of panic attacks, her family (mostly her husband) would often take her to the local insane asylum where she could be subjected to electroshock therapy and even prefrontal lobotomy. This actually happened to my highly creative and intelligent grandmother, who couldn't fit in with Colonial society, constant pregnancy (not all of which survived full term) and used to have 'nervous breakdowns' whereupon she was sent to the 'loony bin' for shock therapy. Fascinatingly, the vibrator was first invented as a treatment for anxiety (sex again)!

In the early and mid-20th century, anxiety was still considered mostly a female condition, although returning soldiers with PTSD were treated with opiates (morphine) and some people were even sterilized. There was a hodgepodge of treatments ranging from opiates, to shock therapy to valium (diazepam). The abuse of tranquilisers (which are highly addictive and frequently prescribed to 'hysterical' women), was brilliantly captured in Jacqueline Susan's 1966 book, The Valley of the Dolls (dolls being a synonym for pills, mostly washed down with Vodka). Freudian psychoanalysis was also very popular in the mid to late 20th Century.

Nowadays, things are much more advanced---or are they? In the latest issue of the DSM (the Diagnostic and Statistical Manual of Mental Disorders (DSM–5)) health anxiety is now known as *two* different 'disorders'; somatic symptom disorder and illness anxiety disorder. In fact, it wasn't even known as health anxiety in the *last* edition of the DSM, and was still called hypochondriasis. The DSM however is subject to multiple criticisms[x], as it 'diagnoses' mental illnesses by listing collections of ill-defined 'symptoms', and tends to diagnose and label as abnormal all sorts of normal conditions, such as grief and childhood tantrums, as mental illness. Therefore, I am going to keep referring to health anxiety as health anxiety…anxiety about one's health.

Perhaps in another 50 years, we will look back on our 2018 fumbling attempts to deal with anxiety with sorrow at how misunderstood the conditions were---or perhaps not. Who knows? Perhaps we will discover a 'physical' cause (of course, any mental state IS physical) and will treat it with a vaccine, a course of psilocybin or a brain re-wiring! Whatever the future, I am certain that we will become more and more accepting and compassionate towards those of us with mental illness, just as we are compassionate and accepting towards those with any other illness, such as diabetes, heart disease or broken limbs.

What is health?

Before talking about health anxiety, we need to discuss the question, 'what is health?' Many of us with health anxiety do not really understand what health actually means. This is particularly important to anxious people, as they are often perfectionists as well.

Good health however is not black and white; we are not *either* perfect or sick. Health is a continuum, and it differs between individuals and is often dependent on sociodemographic characteristics like age, gender and income.

My concept of health at 56 is different to that when I was 26. If I go for a long run now, and my knees hurt, I do not worry. I have an old knee injury (well, not that old, I snapped my Anterior Cruciate Ligament two years ago and haven't bothered having it operated on) and mild arthritis. If I went running at 26 and had bad knee pain, I would likely think there was something wrong other than age, wear and tear (like injury or over training). I'm also anxious about different health conditions than when I was younger (based on what is more likely to kill me now)! I was afraid of pneumonia and rabies as a child in Africa, HIV as a young adult, and cancer as an older adult.

Despite my health anxiety however, I consider myself quite healthy. On the other hand, someone with a chronic condition, such as asthma or diabetes, might consider themselves healthy if they are managing their condition without using their puffer, or their sugar levels remain in the correct zone.

Some people will also make judgements about the health of themselves, or others based on things like weight or colour of skin. For example, it is no longer fashionable to be very suntanned, but when I was growing up in the 1970s, a tanned skin (which can be very unhealthy) was considered to reflect good health. Others assume that an overweight person is unhealthy and a thin one is healthy, whereas the exact opposite might be true.

So health is not just the complete absence of pain, disease, injury or mental distress. It is a much larger concept, which includes your physical, mental and even social health. You can be extremely healthy in one of these; say you are an athlete in top form, yet still have a mental illness, be socially unhealthy and indeed, have a physical illness or injury.

When you describe your health, what do you focus on the most?
- Your physical health?
- Your mental health?
- Your overall wellbeing?

Unhelpful assumptions

Most people with health anxiety have a set of unhelpful assumptions about their health. All of us, whether we like it or not, tend to have a set of largely unwritten rules (values) about how we *should* live our lives. These are often taught to us in early childhood, at school, and through the experiences of life. Mostly, our unwritten rules are quite helpful, and include things like not eating too much junk food, not being cruel to animals and or taking regular exercise. Our rules and values are most helpful when they are true (it is good to get regular exercise) but are still flexible (don't go for a run if we've a fever, or at night in a dangerous place).

However, a tendency of anxious people (and those with the related condition, OCD) is to have *un*helpful and *in*flexible rules; which often originate the same way as our health anxiety. So, an anxious parent who makes a big fuss over the child, even for the slightest illness or injury, may well trigger the same thing in their own child. These then become the largely unconscious rules by which you feel you should live your life: for example, any pain or fever is bad and should be medicated, and if severe, is a symptom of something very serious; or if I ever feel even slightly ill, I should go to the doctor straight away; or if I don't wash my hands after touching an animal, I am bound to get ill.

In the context of health anxiety, this often manifests in the assumption that the only desirable state of health is 100% or perfect health according to our own definition. But, as we saw earlier, health is a relative concept, and means different things to different people. For example, many with chronic, even life threatening illnesses still think that they are healthy. An aspect of this is weight; it is often assumed that if a person is overweight or obese, that they are unhealthy and unfit, and that if someone is thin, that they are healthy and fit. This is complete nonsense, lots of overweight people are extremely healthy, and speaking personally, I've been passed many times in marathons by people twice my size---and twice my speed!

A common characteristic of health anxiety is that **all bodily changes**---any symptoms, lumps, bumps, spots etc.---must be taken seriously, as they could be a sign of a bad illness; they must be investigated by a doctor, and a diagnosis should be given. But no sooner than one symptom or spot turns out to be benign (often after extensive and unnecessary tests) another one is bound to turn up, especially as we age. Doctors are busy people and are concerned about missing something, or being sued, so they will often offer tests, sometimes just to get rid of the patient. Our assumptions are also fed by the media, in that we learn that we need to catch things early or else it will be too late. **These rules are often identified by the words 'should' or 'must'.**

So, what IS Health Anxiety?

It's perfectly normal to worry about our health if we are under stress, or if we are genuinely sick. Unlike the Black Knight (from the Holy Grail) who dismisses even severed limbs as 'just a flesh wound'; if you get a sudden physical symptom, such as chest pains, extremely high fever or uncontrollable bleeding, you'd be silly to ignore your body trying to communicate that something is seriously wrong and not seek emergency medical attention. Health anxiety tends not to manifest in response to obvious symptoms, but to perceived threats and to minor and normal changes in bodily sensations.

Moreover, health anxiety also manifests in response to threats or changes in sensations to *loved ones* as well as yourself. Many parents are almost constantly anxious about the health of their children, particularly when they are very young. When having children, health anxiety sufferers frequently transfer their anxiety from themselves to their children. Then of course, when the children leave home, they go back to being anxious about their own health.

When my children were babies, particularly in the SIDS (Sudden Infant Death Syndrome) risk period up to 6 months, I was constantly terrified that something would happen to them. Because of this, I used to check whether they were breathing all through the night...which used to wake them up, then they would scream, so I'd breastfeed them to calm them down. This became a self-perpetuating habit, and they only slept through the night after I weaned them (around 1 year old). I was permanently exhausted from lack of sleep...which made me more anxious!

As a note, and I will repeat this often, health anxiety is just as much of an anxiety disorder than any other types of anxiety. All too often, people with health anxiety are mocked as hypochondriacs, drama 'queens', attention seekers and neurotics, and we are told that we just need to 'think positively' and it will go away. These attitudes can be very distressing to someone with health anxiety. Why is it that non-anxious people will sympathise with those who are afraid of, say public speaking or snakes, yet mock those who are afraid of ill health? Even people with severe forms of anxiety, such as PTSD and OCD, can be subject to this type of discrimination and contempt.

Anxiety is NOT fun, and people don't CHOOSE to suffer.

As with other types of anxiety, health anxiety is the result of the body's fight, flight or freeze response getting out of whack. What happens is that our rational response to things, such as a new symptom, or some aspect of our bodies, like a lump or bump, is seen as an imminent threat. We then respond with a physical response to the perceived threat, the symptoms of which can and frequently do, mimic the conditions about we are most afraid. Our brains are very good at creating and amplifying existing symptoms.

Also, those suffering from health anxiety are not afraid of the same diseases, and nor do they always feel anxious. Commonly, people with health anxiety tend to fixate on a certain disease, say a certain type of cancer or heart disease, and often are no more afraid of other diseases than someone who doesn't have health anxiety.

These fears can also be situational, and can change with time. Your childhood fears might disappear entirely and be replaced with new fears as you get older. Often, the fear will reflect your environment, and also your age, particularly as some diseases are more common as you get older.

> I first experienced health anxiety when I was quite young, probably around 9, when I was sent to boarding school. Health anxiety is often triggered by traumatic events in childhood, such as being sent away from one's parents, a death in the family or abuse. As a child, I feared tetanus and rabies. These fears were not irrational, however, as we lived in the African bush where rabies was endemic in the wild animal population; and tetanus is common too. Later, I feared meningitis, HIV and still rabies. I was even bitten by a dog in South Africa and insisted on both tetanus and rabies vaccinations--- a lot more painful than the bite. When I came back for the second injection, they asked, 'was it a domestic dog, and is it still alive'. When I answered yes to both, they told me to 'go away'…which exacerbated my anxiety

---

Those with health anxiety may also be totally unafraid of a disease that others are terrified of. This fear may also be irrational (often to the sufferer more than anyone else). I, for example, am afraid of specific types of cancer, but not particularly concerned about cardiovascular disease or dementia. I know that this is irrational, as my family has no history of cancer, and any deaths have been from heart disease, related cardiovascular conditions or dementia. I even have mild arrhythmia and high blood pressure, neither of which cause me the slightest concern. Health anxiety is therefore is not necessarily related to the **actual risk** of contracting an illness. Indeed, it seems to be more common that people are afraid of rare diseases, that they are not at all likely to contract, and not of the more common illnesses. One of the biggest fears discussed on HA forums is that of the extremely rare disease, ALS (Lou Gehrig's disease, of which Stephen Hawking died). I will discuss risk perception later in the book as skewed risk perception is quite significant in health anxiety sufferers.

Health anxiety can also be indirect, where you may not be particularly afraid for your own health, but terribly afraid for the health of one of your family, such as a child, spouse or parent. Thus you may not fear cancer, for example, but something like meningococcal disease, which can rapidly strike young children, and which early symptoms can mimic milder and more common diseases such as the flu.

Some people, and I confess I am one of these, in the absence of any symptoms or sick loved ones (though the loved ones of those with health anxiety soon learn not to tell you if they are ill) will then stress out about the health of other loved ones---your pets! I am hyper aware of any change in my dog's breathing or manner, in case it is a paralysis tick (even though she is on two tick prevention treatments, because why use one when you can use two). But my dog is a Jack Russell cross, and they are the worst sulkers in the canine kingdom, so usually odd behavior is because I'm petting the cat too much, or I haven't given her a treat, or just because it's cold (or hot) and she doesn't like it, no wonder she's named Princess.

One of the most important things to be aware of with health anxiety is that it is a medical condition. Even in the 21st Century, mental illness, sadly, is still subject to stigma, is not taken seriously, is considered less valid than an illness with more physical manifestations, and is even discounted by some medical professionals. Unfortunately, health anxiety, perhaps even more than other mental illnesses, is often mocked by others, with sufferers called hypochondriacs (the original name for health anxiety) or worse. But people with health anxiety can be extremely distressed, and their condition can have severe impacts on their lives, relationships and work.

It's also important to understand that not all symptoms are psychosomatic in origin. Anxiety over physical symptoms or a known illness is perfectly natural; as is anxiety over unexplained symptoms.

There are many stories about people who have a deep concern about a symptom, which has been brushed off by doctors, and which has turned out to a serious disease. Moreover, if you have an illness, particularly a chronic or potentially life-threatening illness, then it is perfectly normal to feel anxious about the disease. If for example, you have had cancer or some other illness and are in remission, it is perfectly understandable to be anxious, often severely anxious, about the possibility of the disease returning.

The more common type of health anxiety however, is when you constantly worry about the possibility of getting or having a life-threatening illness, whether or not you have any symptoms. Alternatively, a minor and normal bodily change might be seen as a symptom of the dread disease. When I was younger and terrified of rabies (even if never bitten or licked by an animal) I was extremely anxious. Unfortunately, anxiety is also a symptom of rabies!

How do you know if you have health anxiety?

You almost certainly know whether you have health anxiety---or at least, others do. Certain unsympathetic friends and family may have always referred to you as a hypochondriac, or when you start talking about your health, they change the subject. Jokes aside, if you answer 'yes' to most of these questions, you likely have health anxiety.

During the past six months:
- "Have you been preoccupied with having a serious illness because of body symptoms, which have lasted at least six months?
- Have you felt distressed due to this preoccupation?
- Have you found that this preoccupation impacts negatively on all areas of life, including family life, social life and work?
- Have you needed to carry out constant self-examination and self-diagnosis?
- Have you experienced disbelief over a diagnosis from a doctor, or felt you are unconvinced by your doctor's reassurances that you are fine?
- Do you constantly need reassurance from doctors, family and friends that you are fine, even if you don't really believe what you are being told?"[xi]

When is health anxiety a cause for concern?

So, as we've seen, a degree of anxiety about your own or a loved one's health is perfectly natural. Only a sociopath or someone unable to feel emotions would, for example, not feel anxious if they had a cancer diagnosis, or a family member was seriously ill. And having regular health checks is important, particularly as we all get older, and certain illnesses become more likely. But when does health anxiety become a problem? When is it a cause for concern?

Health anxiety arises when your concerns:
- "are excessive,
- are out of proportion to the realistic likelihood of having an actual and serious medical problem,
- are persistent despite negative test results and/or reassurance from your health practitioner,
- lead to unhelpful behaviours such as excessive checking, reassurance seeking (e.g., from doctors, family or friends), or avoidance (e.g., of check-ups, doctors, health related information),
- cause you significant distress, or impair your ability to go about your day-to-day life" [xii], and
- are irrational.

Excessive: This is, of course, a subjective term. You might think your concerns are perfectly average, while your partner thinks they are excessive. Generally speaking, if a lot of people tell you that you are excessively concerned about your health, then they are likely correct. I can't read minds (I don't think anyone can) but comparing myself (with health anxiety) to people I know (who don't have health anxiety), *they* do not constantly worry about their health, unless they have an actual symptom. Then they go and get it checked, without dreading that it might be the precursor of something fatal and horrible. They also don't spend hours or longer worrying about their health. They also do not spend hours or more worrying that they *might* get or already have a dread disease, especially if they have no symptoms.

Out of proportion: Reading health anxiety forums is, funny enough, is something that I find helpful to soothe my own anxiety (more on that later). But when reading these, it becomes apparent that people are generally anxious about rare and horrible diseases, and not common diseases, which are much more likely to kill them. I once diagnosed myself with a horrible type of skin cancer, that mostly struck men over 70 with fair skin and depressed immune systems who had spent all their lives working in the sun (none of which apply to me). Doctors have a saying, *'look for horses, not zebras'*; this means that in the vast majority of cases, the most likely cause of your symptoms is what you have, and not something which strikes 0.000000001% of the population. Also, even if you do have something, it is not necessarily going to be fatal (this is catastrophizing, and I discuss it later).

Persistent: Sometimes, if you get a symptom checked out, and the doctor says it is 'nothing', it might reassure you for a time, and then you start worrying again whether the doctor was wrong. I had a lipoma on my leg once, and I saw FIVE doctors---all of whom said, it's a lipoma. I still insisted on getting it cut out, convinced it was sarcoma and found out it was---a lipoma. Now I have a scar, and it's grown back, but this time I'm not worried. The world of medicine is not always so cut and dried. There are many conditions out there that are still relatively unknown, and sometimes doctors just don't know, or judge that what you have is not doing anything, so maybe leave it for a bit. This is terrifying, particularly if it is a low-level tumor or something like that. But modern medicine over-diagnoses many illnesses, and treats many things which are often better left alone.

Unhelpful behaviours: People with health anxiety often exhibit excessive checking behaviour, maybe poking and prodding a suspicious spot or lump hundreds of times a day. This just makes the lump tender---and you worry more. Unhelpful behaviours also include excessive doctor visits; if you don't like what the first doctor says, then better get it checked out by another. If you are lucky enough to live somewhere with accessible and not too expensive medical services, like Australia, then it's easy to go to repeated doctors. But this puts a huge pressure on the medical system, with doctors having to constantly reassure patients who have nothing wrong with them, and possibly causing sicker people to miss out. Emergency ward visits are an extreme of this; and may even lead to the death of someone with a real heart attack and not just indigestion (still, go straight to emergency if you have chest pain!).

Conversely, another unhelpful behavior characteristic of health anxiety is **avoidance.** This may sound contradictory, but people with health anxiety often go between two extremes; frequent doctor visits---and complete avoidance of doctors or anything medical related. This may even extend to avoiding watching certain programs on TV, not reading anything about the disease or even not driving or walking past a hospital. I tend to do this around regular testing; in Australia we've government sponsored mammograms for women over 50, and I am always a year or more late for these, because I am terrified that they might find something---but then the more I put it off, the more anxious I get! Sometimes I avoid one type of test and do another, or I go to the doctor for one condition, in the hope that s/he will ask me about the 'real' problem. **Distress:** Let's be straight now; health anxiety can cause huge amounts of stress, worry and even trauma. If you are in the throes of a health anxiety episode, this can take up huge amounts of your, cause you to go around constantly feeling dread, nausea, faint, hyperventilating, panic attacks and other horrible emotional feelings. These can also be, unfortunately, symptoms of diseases, so it's a vicious circle. When I'm going through an episode, I can't eat, so I lose heaps of weight really quickly, then I think I've got late stage cancer because, um, rapid weight loss. Also, you worry all the time, so you can't sleep, then you feel terrible from lack of sleep, and your work and personal life suffers. Health anxiety is horrible.

Irrational: When you are in the throes of a health anxiety episode, your higher, logical brain *knows* that your fears are likely groundless, but it does little to help your obsessive thoughts. I am an academic and have a PhD, and no matter how much I tell myself that my fear de jour is irrational, it makes little difference.

	Never	At times	Often	Always
I worry about my health	0	1	2	3
I worry that I have or may develop a serious health problem	0	1	2	3
I worry that bodily sensations/changes are a sign of a serious medical problem	0	1	2	3
I find it difficult to control or let go of my health worries	0	1	2	3
I mentally scan my body/and or mind for signs that something is wrong	0	1	2	3
I focus my attention on my bodily sensations or symptoms	0	1	2	3
I physically check my body for symptoms or changes	0	1	2	3
I frequently visit health professionals (i.e. GPs, specialists) to discuss my health concerns and symptoms, or to have tests performed	0	1	2	3
I avoid health professionals (i.e. GPs, specialists) as I am too worried about my health and/or test results	0	1	2	3
I have continued to worry about my health despite my doctor's reassurance or despite negative tests	0	1	2	3
I discuss my symptoms with my family and/or friends	0	1	2	3
I avoid people, places or activities that trigger off health worries	0	1	2	3
I avoid people, places or activities that trigger off particular physical sensations	0	1	2	3

Adapted from CCI (Score: 0 – 13 Low; 14 – 25 Medium; 26 - 39 High)

Negative impacts of health anxiety

So, as we've seen, health anxiety is much more than simple worrying about your health. Furthermore, it can also have **negative impacts on your physical, mental and emotional health**! Oh dear, we can't win whatever we do. We worry about getting sick and then the worry makes us sick! So let's jump right in and explore all the negativity---then we will concentrate on the better stuff---positive things that work!

Physical Impacts: Because this book is about health anxiety, I will start with health. Anxiety is bad for our health. Firstly, anxiety gives rise to horrible actual symptoms, like palpitations, nausea, cold sweats, hot flushes, headache, lack of sleep, light-headedness, dizziness, muscle pain and spasm, backache, gut problems, cramping, gas, diarrhea, tingling, detachment, etc. As if you didn't have enough to worry about! Many of these are what doctors call psychosomatic, or somatiform pain[xiii] which in itself can be a disorder (at least, according to the DSM 5---although this tends to label almost all human behaviour as some sort of disorder.

Unfortunately, anxiety, including health anxiety, can also have real health impacts[xiv]. Anxiety has been linked to heart disease, chronic respiratory disorders, irritable bowel syndrome, an overworked nervous system, depressed immune system and greater susceptibility to ulcers. When we are stressed, levels of cortisol (a stress hormone) rise, increasing heart rate, blood pressure and using more energy for the body to respond. Chronic stress keeps cortisol (and adrenaline, the 'fight or flight' hormone) levels artificially raised. This is discussed further in the section on the origins of health anxiety.

Anxiety also has indirect impacts that affect our health. For example, we may self-medicate with alcohol, tobacco or other drugs, and these may have severe health impacts. We may also turn to over eating, eating junk food or too much coffee or soft drinks.

When in the middle of an anxiety attack, we may neglect our fitness regimes in case they exacerbate the symptoms. Anxiety also directly influences the gut and many find that they have diarrhea or IBS (irritable bowel syndrome) when anxious (this is common, just go into the toilets before a marathon for evidence). Finally, anxiety affects our sleep, and poor sleep has been linked to everything from obesity to depression to anxiety!

Psychological Impacts: Ok, now that we are nice and depressed, let's talk about some of the psychological impacts of anxiety. A good place to start with is depression. Depression and anxiety are best friends, they go hand in hand, with many people having both disorders. Other mental health conditions that are often linked with anxiety are Obsessive Compulsive Disorder (OCD), phobias and panic disorder (of course), ADD, eating disorders and substance abuse. Many also use substances such as alcohol or other drugs to help ease the symptoms of anxiety. Unfortunately, while it is effective in the (very) short term, alcohol is a depressant and frequently makes anxiety worse. Also it causes cancer[xv].

Social impacts: Anxiety can have serious effects on our relationships, with intimate relationships such as with partners, but also with children, friends, other family and colleagues. If you are constantly worrying about your health, it is difficult for you to connect with other people, to listen to their conversation and to engage in social activities. If you are 'good' at communicating your worries, then you may also cause your loved ones to worry (though they tend to stop worrying after the 7th 'heart attack' of the month, and get annoyed with you). If on the other hand, like many health anxiety suffers, you are embarrassed about your worries and you hide them from your loved ones, they still pick it up, and worry about what is wrong with you that you won't talk about. And in my experience, things unknown are always imagined as way worse than they really are. You also might find yourself avoiding people who ask too many questions, or getting irritated with others who are impatient with your health concerns.

Work impacts: Spending hours worrying about your health impacts your work, and your productivity. If you are spending half your work day Googling your symptoms or your feared disease, you are not being very productive. Taking lots of sick days and spending time at doctors and specialists also impacts your work. Even if you are not doing any of these things, and are just worrying; it is very difficult to concentrate, and the lack of sleep and inconsistent diet that is common in an anxiety episode, only makes things worse. Even if no-one says anything at work, you may get a reputation for taking fake 'sickies' all the time and being a slacker.

General wellbeing: It is difficult to enjoy life if you are constantly worrying about what might happen in the future. We are bad enough at not being in the moment and taking time to enjoy the present, but anxiety makes this ten times worse. Everything reminds us of what we are terrified of, and it is incredibly difficult to take joy in anything. Tara Brach, my favourite speaker, likens this to having anticipated attending a beautiful symphony for months, being so excited, then when you get there, you realise that you have left the back door open---and you cannot leave! How much enjoyment and attention do you give the concert?

Another way that anxiety effects our wellbeing is that when we are in the throes of an anxiety episode, we frequently neglect our healthy lifestyle efforts. We may not eat enough fruit and vegetables, or snack on sweets or junk food, or binge eat. We may also neglect our exercise routines, not go for walks even, or avoid the gym. When I had a 'horrible lump' on my ankle, I wore socks everywhere, and wouldn't go swimming in case someone noticed it, and asked me what it was (it was about 2mm in diameter, and turned out to be an infected splinter!) Of course, when we neglect our normal healthy lifestyle because we are so stressed that we are feeling sick, then we feel worse!

Relationships with medical professionals: Like the little boy who cried wolf, doctors figure out very quickly that we've health anxiety. This is also the origin of the title of this book. I have a very sympathetic doctor (really) and when I saw her for about the 3rd time in a month, with suspected 'liver cancer' (aka delayed muscle pain from the gym and poor posture at my desk), she asked me, "what are you dying from this week?"

Unfortunately some doctors are not quite as sympathetic, and will brush off your concerns, and when you visit them with something that might not be health anxiety, might even ignore or brush aside a genuine problem, which is the last thing you want.

Financial impacts: Health anxiety is expensive, and extremely so in countries without subsidized health care, like the USA. Even in Australia, you are not going to get much attention from a bulk-billing doctor (subsidized by Medicare), as they are extremely busy; so you are likely going to have to go to a fee-paying doctor. Also, doctors do mean well, despite what some people think, and they don't want to send you away without finding what is wrong with you, so they often schedule unnecessary tests and scans (all of which can be very expensive).

I snapped my Anterior Cruciate Ligament (ACL) last year, and got a MRI for free, but when it was still hurting, they wouldn't give me another one for free until a year had passed. Rather than pay the fee, I just ignored the pain, and worked on my physio's exercises, and it got better on its own (maybe because I actually listened to my physio and cut back on running and yoga). Often too, doctors will prescribe you pills and potions, and these can also be expensive, have side effects and will make you feel sick.

So, obviously health anxiety isn't pleasant and no-one knows that better than someone who has the problem. It's got nothing to do with rational thinking or intelligence or income or anything; it can hit anyone. So, how does health anxiety develop? Why do some people get it and not others?

CHAPTER TWO: ORIGINS OF HEALTH ANXIETY

How Health Anxiety develops

Anxiety is the most common mental illness, but of course, health anxiety does not strike everyone. There are multiple, interconnected reasons why a person has health anxiety and another does not. Most medical professionals don't know the reason why some people are anxious and some are not, but some common characteristics predispose certain people to develop the disorder. Pretty much it comes down to nature, nurture or both; so let's start by blaming our parents (nature *and* nurture).

Parental modelling

One of the commonest origins of health anxiety is because a significant other (often a parent or sibling) also has health anxiety. My mother for example, has, as long as I have known her (56 years) been convinced that she has cancer. She is terrified of the disease. When I was young, I was quite a sickly child, as I had frequent tonsillitis, and she used to fuss so much over me, that whenever she wanted to feel my forehead to see if I had a fever, I would run away, and pretend not to be sick even if I was. Most of my family have varying degrees of anxiety, although not all have health anxiety. Genetically, I had no chance!

Another causal factor is when a significant other has suffered or died from a serious illness. This is particularly important at certain life stages, such as childhood or adolescence. It is relatively common that health anxiety develops in response to someone having a long term chronic illness. Watching a person that you love (especially a parent) suffer over a long period is extremely distressing, particularly if you feel that you are helpless and cannot do anything for them. Some people find that their health anxiety is triggered by others talking about a dread disease, seeing something on TV or on the internet or learning of someone with a terminal illness (even strangers).

Another related stressor is the death of a close family member, even if it was sudden. Children often have little comprehension about mortality, and when the fact that people are *not* immortal and not going to be there forever suddenly hits them, it can be a terrible shock, and precipitate a number of future problems. The child may then perceive themselves to be very vulnerable. This can also happen with the death of non-humans, such as a beloved pet.

> We used to go on holiday every year, and I was always happy to come home, to see my pets and sleep in my own bed. One year when I was about 8, we came home to find that all our dogs (except one) had been stung to death by bees, including a puppy that we'd raised from 2 days old. This was a terrible shock, and still affects me. Now, when I go away, which I force myself to do (and enjoy) I always have a nagging dread that I'm going to come home to something wrong, horrible and unexpected.

Wanting to stay in control and almost to 'know' the future is characteristic of health anxiety.

Being ill yourself

Having had a serious or long term illness yourself can predispose you to health anxiety. This is particularly the case for illnesses such as cancer; many people who have beaten cancer and are in remission, but live with fear that the disease will return. This is not helped by the media reporting on celebrities with similar illnesses. Moreover, if we've been seriously ill, we are likely to be more attuned to the sensations of our body and any changes we might notice. Doctors too are very risk averse, and will frequently tell people of all the possible complications, risks and chances of recurrence, which may lead to increased fear. Medical jargon does not help in this regard, as some terms sound much more serious than they really are; for example, the medical term for bruising is a traumatic hematoma, which sounds very ominous.

Genetics and epigenetics

Related to parental modelling (nurture), nature also has a major part to play in the development of health anxiety. Indeed, most researchers acknowledge that genetics plays a significant part in all anxiety disorders[i]. Researchers have investigated identical twins[ii] (who have identical genes) and other related people, and have found an increased risk of many anxiety disorders and related issues, such as phobic and panic disorder, OCD and PTSD, if family members also suffer from these. For example, there is a 5-16% increase in the risk of panic disorder if a first degree family member (parent or sibling) also has panic disorder.

So what about epigenetics? Indeed, what *is* epigenetics? This is one of those terms like quantum mechanics that is bandied around, but most of us are pretty clueless on what it means[iii]. Basically, we are all born with a specific and mostly unique genetic makeup (unless we are an identical twin or a clone). Epigenetics refers to something that can turn a gene on or off; a 'marker' that is on top of a gene that tells it to express in a certain way or not. Very simply, epigenetic markers can change how the same genetic sequence is expressed. Normal mice that are born with methylated gene 'agouti' are skinny and brown, but if this gene is un-methylated by giving the pregnant mother BPA (Bisphenol A, a plastic additive), then babies born are yellow and fat---*despite* being genetically identical.

What is really interesting is that epigenetics can influence the behavior of children and even grandchildren because of past trauma. Many of us nowadays have had family members who were in various wars, and their experiences could have contributed to our anxiety. Likewise, our experiences, say of childhood or domestic abuse could have affected our children and grandchildren. The experiences of famine, for example, have been passed down to at least three generations. The negative epigenetic effects of early trauma can be reversed by living in a low stress environment, or (potentially) by chemically fixing the aberrant DNA[iv].

DNA comprises four nucleotides, C (Cytosine), G (Guanine), T (Thymine) and A (Adenine). DNA methylation means that a methyl group (CH3) is added to the DNA (usually to the Cytosine atom). Methylation is common in mammals and vital to healthy growth and development, and suppresses potentially dangerous sequences of DNA (such as cancer mutations). Methylation can be reversed (de/un-methylated) by chemical or laboratory processes, by cancers, and **by trauma**. [v]

Evolutionary biology – fight, flight or freeze

From an evolutionary biology perspective, humans have evolved a response to danger known at the 'fight, flight or freeze reflex' (as discussed earlier). When we were naked vulnerable creatures roaming the African savannah, if something threatened us, we could respond in one of three ways: if we perceived ourselves as stronger, we could fight; if we perceived ourselves as weaker, we could run away (flight); and if the threat was so great that we could do nothing, we could freeze.

Implicated in all of these behaviours are various stress hormones that the amygdala (part of the brain) releases to help us survive. The physiological reactions that happen when we feel threatened (anxious) are designed to help us deal with **physical threats**. These include a spike in blood sugar levels from increased cortisol in the bloodstream, a redistribution of blood flow around the body, tense muscles, dry mouth and a more active spleen. If we were to choose flight (not fully consciously) we feel a rush of adrenaline or cortisol, which helps us run faster from danger.

However, we've long since moved from being vulnerable mammals to the strongest (and most destructive) creatures on earth. But while our society has rapidly evolved, our bodies haven't and our brains still preserve our primitive fear responses. The only problem is, anxious people are have overly sensitive fight-flight-freeze mechanisms, and their chemical reactions are on permanent hyper alter to non-threatening, everyday things like commuting, office politics, other politics, too much work pressure---and worrying about our health. None of these are life-threatening, at least in the short term, but the cumulative effect of these stress hormones definitely can damage our health.

One positive is that if we've hyper vigilant fear mechanisms, our ancestors were pretty clever and good at surviving. The fearless and stupid ones got eaten by saber-toothed tigers or fell off cliffs. Unfortunately, nowadays, there are few man eating carnivores lurking in the shrubbery, and if we are foolhardy enough to go free climbing or base jumping (unlikely in anxious people), then we are responsible for our own demise. But no-one told our bodies that. We still have a bit of evolving to do.

But despite our super-powered fear mechanisms giving us evolutionary advantages, they also make us highly sensitive about our health. Instead of saber-toothed tigers, we are frequently focused on threats (illness) and means by which we can escape the threat (going to the doctor or constant checking). It is difficult to enjoy the concert (life around us) if we are constantly worrying. This sensitivity also manifests in slight changes in our body, minor pains, lumps and bumps and spots. Because we are hypersensitive to threats; any change, no matter how minor, can seem a huge problem. People with health anxiety are ultra-sensitive to changes that most people would not even notice.

But when we are constantly afraid and hyper-vigilant, we pay so much attention to the symptom (threat) that it becomes (in our mind) much larger and more serious than it actually is. We also start to lose our sense of reality, that the constant checking for changes or growth, and poking and prodding, we don't even know if it's getting worse or not, and cannot remember even what it looked like five minutes ago. What I thought was a huge unsightly lump on my ankle, so much so that I wore socks all the time so no-one could see it, was in reality, about 2mm wide, and the only way even I could see it clearly was to look at it under a bright light, through a magnifying glass. Of course, when it turned out *not* to be cancer, I never bothered to look at it again, and completely forgot about it.

Trauma

As we've seen, parental or even more removed relatives can pass on trauma through epigenetics. However, a major contributing factor to anxiety and health anxiety is personal trauma, the most serious manifestation of which is Post Traumatic Stress Disorder (PTSD). PTSD is an extreme form of anxiety and depression that people who have been exposed to things such as war, rape, domestic or other violence, death of a loved one, assault and other trauma. It can result in flashbacks, nightmares, phobias and problems with relationships and work.

Health anxiety can result from the same or similar causes as PTSD, and even by less extreme forms of violence, abuse or the like. These traumas remind us of how vulnerable we really so we may project the vulnerability inwards, and feel constantly threatened. Many of the treatments for PTSD are the same as treatments for anxiety.

We also may not even know that we've been exposed to trauma; and that certain things in our past would be considered traumatic. I literally had an argument with a therapist once, because he said that in a previous violent relationship, where I had been at times, afraid for my own and children's' lives, was trauma. Nonsense! I said, stating that it had been many years in the past, and had long forgiven him. Of course, it was trauma.

Gut bacteria

Fascinating new research shows that gut bacteria---hence the food we eat---may contribute to anxiety. An 'unhealthy' gut biome could be linked to greater levels of anxiety, and also to other mental illness, such as depression. Our gut biome (total bacterial environment) can be impacted by common things, such as a poor diet, antibiotics and even a lack of fiber. Researchers at Oxford found that subjects given prebiotics had lower levels of anxiety and the stress hormone cortisol[vi]. Anecdotally, some say that if they eat too much junk food, drink too much alcohol, or give up (or take up) eating meat, then their anxiety worsens.

> This is also another dimension of epigenetics; a short sequence of nucleotide called miRNA controls how some genes are expressed, and miRNAs in the amygdala are linked with anxiety. The health of our gut microbiome has been shown (in mice) to influence miRNA in the brain, with mice with poor microbiomes having differing levels of the compound, and thus anxiety[vii].

Risk perception

Another contributing factor to health anxiety (and other types of anxiety) is misunderstanding of or the inability to understand true risk. The best example of this is the difference between flying and driving. Many of us are, to some extent, afraid of flying, yet get in our cars every day without a second thought. But the risk of being injured or dying in a car crash are far higher than being in a plane crash. In fact, aeroplanes are the SAFEST form of mass transit, and in the USA, you have a 1:112 lifetime chance of dying in motor vehicle crash (1-112) and a 1:96,566 lifetime chance of dying in a plane crash[viii].

Similarly, many overestimate the chances of extremely unlikely events happening to them, such as shark attacks (1:11,500,000), terrorist incidents (1:45,000) and earthquakes (1:130,000); and underestimate the chances of common events, such as falling (1:133), walking (1:672) and---I'm reluctant to put this in a book on health anxiety, but---heart disease and cancer (1:7)[ix].

Time orientation and health anxiety

Time perspective? What on earth has that got to do with health anxiety? Quite a lot it seems. A well-known psychologist and researcher, Phillip Zimbardo, has devised a theory that people have different time perspectives, or how individuals divide their experience and decision-making into time categories[x]. For some, the present is everything, they make a decision based on the here and now.

So the decision 'should I go for a run' is based on how they feel at that moment, and most likely, the weather. For others, the past dictates how they behave and make decisions, so if they think, 'should I go for a run', they might think of the past pleasurable runs or possibly, how tired they got the last time they tried running. Yet others are future-oriented, and when deciding whether to go for a run, will think, 'it's raining, but if I go for a run, I will feel good afterwards, and it will help me maintain my weight'.

These time categories have further sub-categories[xi][xii] such as past-positive (good memories of the past), past-negative (bad memories), present hedonistic (live in the moment, seeking pleasure), present fatalistic (fatalistic, predetermined), future-oriented (planning for the future) and transcendental future-oriented (rewarded in the afterlife).

Ok, but health anxiety! Well, funny enough, future oriented people are not necessarily more anxious about potential health threats. Indeed, present fatalistic and past negative people are more prone to anxiety in general (research has only really focused on GAD however, so this research may be lesser relevant to health anxiety)[xiii].

But this result does concur with some of the origins of health anxiety, such as parental modelling, trauma, past illness and indeed, epi/genetics. All of these are past negative, and are highly influential in whether anxiety develops or not[xiv].

The media and the internet.

The health anxiety mantra should be 'NEVER EVER GOOGLE YOUR SYMPTOMS!'

We've almost constant access to news about health, and information. No longer do we've to go to the library and find some huge, heavy and complicated textbook to look up our symptoms. Unfortunately, the media will not sell stories if they are boring, so they love to exaggerate things to make them more newsworthy. Also, most journalists do not understand scientific subjects, are unable to read research papers, and report these incorrectly. How many 'cures for cancer' have you read about this week? If you read the actual journal article, it is almost always research done on mice or even fruit flies, or in a petri dish, and human trials haven't started.

Also, the media tend to report on rare and incurable diseases, and fatal diseases; and because these are often reported, it appears that they are more common than they actually are (see Risk Perception). It is like buying a new yellow car; all of a sudden, you see hundreds of yellow cars that you never noticed before. So, when the media starts a story on a rare form of skin cancer, then your own (benign) skin lesions start looking suspicious. Even trained medical specialists sometimes have problems visually detecting certain skin cancers, which is why they biopsy suspicious lesions. A lay person such as you or me is almost certainly wrong.

Another thing the media likes to do is report on misdiagnosed diseases; with stories of patients repeatedly going to doctors, told that there was nothing wrong, and then finding that they had something horrible, that could have been cured if they had found it earlier. Sure, this does happen, but very rarely. They also report, often completely incorrectly, on the side effects of certain medications, so much so that people will stop taking lifesaving medications.

For example, in 2015, a respected Australian media program ran a highly negative story about statin drugs (used to treat high cholesterol in people at risk for heart attacks) with the result that nearly 70,000 people stopped taking these drugs[xv]. Indeed, these drugs are often overprescribed, and have some negative side-effects; but they also save people's lives by lowering inflammation and reduce risk of narrowed arteries[xvi].

Then there's the internet. The first commandment of health anxiety is to NEVER CONSULT DOCTOR GOOGLE. For example, research showed that headaches may be a symptom of a brain tumour in about 0.00005% of people, yet if you look up headache on Google, you get brain tumour as the most common result in about 50% of cases. I couldn't even find the original research, because the first two pages of search results were ALL about brain cancer! Just goes to show (and that is not the filter bubble as I never Google symptoms, and brain cancer is not one of my health anxiety triggers, as I am so terrified of it, that I am too afraid to even *think* about it). There are hundreds of memes about the popular health site, WebMD, with captions like, *'something that makes a mild cold into a deadly disease that will kill you in the next 24 hours'*; and *'according to WebMD, my symptoms mean I died 3 years ago'*. Never Google (yes, we all do it).

Negatives of society

Globally, the incidence of all types of anxiety, depression and many other mental illnesses continues to rise. Depression used to be mostly confined to the elderly, but now it is a disease of youth; and the incidence is 10 to 20 times higher than 50 years ago. Certainly, this is partly due to changes in diagnosis as well as the development of certain pharmaceuticals (and the incentives given to medical professionals to prescribe these); but it is my opinion (and many others) that it is also due to the type of society in which we live.

Firstly, we are working longer hours to pay our bills, especially housing, the price of which has risen exponentially in past decades. For example, housing in all Australian major centers (home to nearly 90% of the population) is rated as severely or extremely unaffordable. Moreover, jobs nowadays are more insecure than ever, with constant pressure to perform or be laid off. Both parents usually work and if they take time off for maternity or paternity leave, it is usually for a very short period. Long vacations have also disappeared, and many people take no vacations at all.

We've also lost our connection to a spiritual purpose. Religion used to play a major part in society, providing community, a source of help and advice. Arguably, people need to have some sort of faith or sense of purpose in life, not to feel that they are just on an endless treadmill to pay the bills and die. We've lost respect (justifiably in many cases) for our institutions; be those the churches and the priests, the government and even scientists.

We've also, particularly in the last decade, become increasingly 'plugged in' to the matrix of the internet and social media. We are constantly bombarded with clever psychological techniques to keep us addicted, to keep us checking our phones and our email and our social media. We cannot escape work anywhere, and people literally suffer mental distress if they are in a place with no connection to the internet or telephone networks. Social media also makes us increasingly insecure and fearful; we are bombarded with visions of people's 'perfect' lives as well as online fear-mongering. We are losing the ability to differentiate between what is real or fake.

As an example, I had a friend staying over one night, and just as I had dropped off to sleep, he knocked on my door, saying wake up, and I must listen to something. He was playing a radio broadcast on his IPad, sent as a Facebook link from his brother, which sounded like Russia and NATO had started a conflict, and it was escalating so much that nuclear weapons were being launched. It turned out to be fake, a scenario created to raise awareness on the proliferation of nuclear weapons, but it was incredibly realistic. I was absolutely convinced, and it was only when I looked up reliable media sources, did I start getting suspicious. Still, to me it felt almost the same viscerally, as when I heard about September 11 or other world disasters; no difference between reality and fiction.

As we've shown, anxiety and health anxiety have many origins, and most of us who suffer from health anxiety probably have other forms of anxiety, and can tick a number of different causes. It is a complex situation, and it is NOT OUR FAULT (well, of course it isn't, but it is always useful to emphasize that). In Buddhism, they speak of the 'second arrow': "...*any time we suffer misfortune, two arrows fly our way. The first arrow, the pain, is the actual bad event. The second arrow, the suffering, is our reaction to the bad event, the way we chose to respond emotionally. The first arrow often is unavoidable. The second arrow often is self-inflicted. Avoiding the second arrow requires mature emotional awareness.*"[xvii][xviii]

We may be suffering, but it is **not our fault;** and we should not beat ourselves up about it; and nor should we've to put up with people making fun of it. Because it is anything but funny.

CHAPTER THREE: WHAT TRIGGERS HEALTH ANXIETY?

Not all of us have health anxiety all the time, though an unfortunate few do. I have health anxiety in bursts, triggered by external (or internal) stressors in my life, and unexplained symptoms. When I don't have health anxiety, my frame of mind in an episode is completely alien to me; I find it difficult to reconcile my non-anxious self with my anxious self. This is not to say that I don't have other types of anxiety, I do; but I definitely have episodic health anxiety. But even those of us who have health anxiety most of the time, will likely find that it is worse at some times than others. So what are some of the things that trigger health anxiety?

TRIGGERS

Someone being diagnosed or dying from a serious illness.

Many of people with health anxiety have a specific disease, or type of disease that they are most afraid of. Usually it is common diseases, such as cancer, but it may also be a specific cancer, or even a very rare disease. Personally, if someone I know is diagnosed with, or worse, dies from cancer, then I know I run the risk of having an episode of health anxiety. For example, I was never particularly afraid of breast cancer, as my health anxiety is more biased towards melanoma and internal organ cancers, but when two people I knew well were not only diagnosed, but eventually died from breast cancer---and I hadn't had my regular mammogram, this precipitated me into first a frenzy of checking, and then not checking---in case I found anything! For some, even reading about or watching a story on TV about *anyone* with a certain disease, say a celebrity, can trigger an anxiety attack.

Medical checkups

When I am due for a regular checkup, say a pap smear or mammogram or my annual skin check, I start becoming anxious in case they find anything. Now, of course, rationally, it is good that I have these checkups, so that if they do find something, it is likely to be caught early, but I am terrified of the uncertainty---even though I have not, in the past year or so since the last one, given it any thought at all. Medical checkups are even worse if you have some symptom, and you want it checked out. I usually present with high blood pressure because I am so terrified of going to the doctor that I'm almost having a panic attack. My doctors don't even take my blood pressure anymore, they just get the nurse to do it (then it's always normal). Also, I find it difficult to actually tell the doctor why I am there, and sometimes have been to a doctor to get something checked out, and have been too afraid to even tell the doctor! So, I might go to the doctor with something that I know is not a symptom of anything fatal (like knee pain from an old injury) and then subtly mention the *other* symptom. Doctors aren't psychics!

Other stress in your life

Stress is a notorious trigger of health anxiety. If you are under stress from work or relationships, or money---or anything really, it makes you more vulnerable to an episode. Stress can also trigger an episode long after the stressor has gone. While you are dealing with the stress, you are busy with all that entails, the pressure and difficult emotions etc. A few weeks or months after a stressful period however (whether this is to do with work, money, relationships, etc.), then a health anxiety relapse is more likely. It's a delayed reaction to the stress and inflammation that it causes in the body.

Of course, stress is an individual thing, and what stresses one person, has no effect on another. There's a much quoted list of the most stressful things in life, and public speaking always seems to be near the top. There's a joke, *"they say people are more afraid of public speaking than they are of snakes. It doesn't seem to make sense. I mean, you don't see someone walking through the desert, suddenly shouting, "Watch out! A podium*! ~Unknown. Of course, many people, myself included, are not in the slightest bit afraid of public speaking (nor am I afraid of snakes), but they are afraid of other things (I won't stand near the edge of any cliff, even if there is a barrier) and some even have phobias about certain objects or circumstances.

So stress depends on the individual person and their circumstances; if you only move house a couple of times a lifetime, it will be extremely stressful; but if you move every year or so, or live in a caravan, moving house most likely won't be particularly stressful. Same with other highly stressful (to some) events, for example, a mutually agreed, amicable separation is a lot less stressful than a contested divorce.

Hormonal changes

Hormonal changes are not discussed often as triggers for anxiety, but many (women in particular) find that their anxiety (health or other forms of anxiety) is worse when they are premenstrual, pregnant or going through menopause. Some researchers even think than certain manifestations of some mental illnesses are primarily hormonal in nature, and that stabilizing hormones such as estrogen and progesterone can also stabilize emotions. A very good friend of mine, Gill, had such extreme mood swings from PMT and then peri-menopause, that she was diagnosed with Bipolar syndrome and prescribed all sorts of pharmaceutical drugs. When younger, the birth control pill moderated the mood swings, and when she transitioned through menopause, her symptoms largely disappeared. Unfortunately, she is still having to withdraw slowly from the mood stabilizers, anti-depressant and anti-psychotic drugs.

Menopause and peri-menopause are particular times that women notice that their anxiety increases; and this is likely linked to emotions as well as hormonal changes[i]. Many researchers have found that anxiety and depressive disorders become worse around menopause, with often the first onset of panic attacks at this stage of life. This was certainly the case for me; my anxiety was at its worst around peri-menopause. One reason why anxiety is so marked then, is that Progesterone---known as the 'calming hormone'---fluctuates wildly around menopause, and low levels also impact sleep quality. Estrogen deprivation can also cause the blood vessels of the brain to constrict, depriving the brain of blood and making us feel woozy and hazy.

Menopause is also a time when women frequently experience other external life stressors; it is a time when they may have both teenage children as well as elderly, sometimes dependent parents. This is known as the 'sandwich generation', where not only are women sandwiched between the generations, but are often coping with other pressures such as relationship problems (their partners, if male, going through their own mid-life crises), and work and money stress. On top of that, there's the emotional overlay of feeling that you are getting older, losing your sexuality and attractiveness, and the all too common weight gain of peri/menopause. That makes a 'perfect storm' for middle aged women. Little wonder for some of them, their anxiety goes through the roof.

Moreover, not just sex hormones influence anxiety, but also stress hormones (such as cortisol etc.) and thyroid hormones. Indeed, fluctuating thyroid hormones are one of the major chemical causes of anxiety, one reason why doctors will often first schedule a thyroid hormone test when a patient presents with anxiety.

Always **check your hormone levels if you suddenly start getting anxious---before going on psychiatric drugs.**

Change in diet

Nowadays, with the trends towards healthy and clean eating, many people drastically change their diets, for example, giving up gluten and wheat products, becoming vegetarian or vegan, cutting out dairy, etc. Mostly, these changes are positive, and will benefit health---particularly if the previous diet was poor. However, dramatic changes in diet can also be detrimental to your health particularly if you follow the latest diet craze on the internet.

For example, even though vegetarianism is healthy, a number of people say that if they change to a plant-based diet too rapidly, that this can exacerbate their anxiety. For myself, I am largely a vegetarian (though I eat dairy) but I have to eat animal protein every now and again otherwise I start becoming more anxious.

The findings of some recent research indicate that anxiety can be fueled by a diet with too much junk food, sugar, coffee and even dairy products (and alcohol of course, but that has its own section). If you are not getting enough nutrients from your diet, especially from fruit, vegetables, lean fats and complex carbohydrates, then this can exacerbate anxiety. B Vitamins in particular are strongly linked to anxiety, and if you are low in these, then this may trigger anxiety. Omega rich foods like oily fish, cultures such as yoghurt, kombucha or kimchi, and high protein foods can all help anxiety. And it goes without saying that too much coffee or caffeine rich foods can make you feel more anxious.

Alcohol (and drugs)

A major trigger of health anxiety is substance abuse, or even just too much 'substance' even if not actually abused. Alcohol is a central nervous system depressant, and while it makes you feel better in the short term, in the long term, it can make you depressed and anxious. One way it does this is by interfering with sleep. For the first half of the night alcohol actually makes you sleep deeper, but then in the second half of the night, when the dehydration and headaches kick in, it makes you feel much worse, so you don't sleep well and miss out on valuable REM sleep. Poor sleep has been linked to many disorders, including obesity and depression!

Alcohol generally has significant impacts on anxiety (amongst other mental health issues). This is often a two way relationship, as mental health issues can also lead to alcohol abuse, often as a 'quick fix' for feeling bad. But although a drink or more makes you feel better in the short term, in the long term, it is a depressant, and makes you feel worse. You may well feel less stressed after a drink or two, but soon you need more to feel the same effect.

Alcohol impacts on brain chemistry, such as levels of serotonin. It is widely accepted that abnormal levels of brain neurotransmitters (chemicals) such as serotonin, are often responsible for many cases of depression, anxiety and OCD. This is why a common treatment for such conditions are various types of SSRI (selective serotonin reuptake inhibitor) drugs such as Zoloft, Prozac and Cipramil, which aim to normalise serotonin levels in the brain. These drugs are not without their side effects (both during taking them, and in withdrawal), which can be quite severe, but are effective for many. On the other hand, if giving up alcohol can achieve similar results, with only positive side effects, then it seems a better choice.

Alcohol is often used to reduce stress, but in the long term, it increases stress. Many chronic drinkers or alcoholics have experienced significant stress in their lives, particularly in childhood, and frequently report that they began drinking to ease the stress. But alcohol is toxic to the body, and drinking above moderate levels, increases physical stress on organs such as the heart, liver and brain. It is also a Group 1 carcinogen (known cause of cancer). [1][ii]

Using alcohol as a stress reducer does not teach coping skills or increase resilience and it can raise cortisol levels – thus creating more stress. When stressed, cortisol levels rise, increasing heart rate, blood pressure and using more energy for the body to respond. Chronic stress keeps cortisol (and adrenaline, the 'fight or flight' hormone) levels artificially raised, and drinking to reduce stress, in the long term, has the opposite effect. Interestingly, because alcohol is often used as a Band-Aid solution for extreme stressors, its impact on cortisol levels exacerbates the habitual nature of drinking,

- [1] *Group 1: Carcinogenic to humans*
- *Group 2A: Probably carcinogenic to humans*
- *Group 2B: Possibly carcinogenic to humans*
- *Group 3: Unclassifiable as to carcinogenicity in humans*
- *Group 4: Probably not carcinogenic to humans*

as cortisol is also linked to habit formation.

Excessive alcohol use is implicated in other serious mental health problems, such as suicide, self-harm and psychosis. Because alcohol reduces inhibitions, it may trigger a self-harm or suicide attempt, which may not have occurred if a person were sober. Its role in reducing inhibitions can also result in behaviour that can have long term impacts on mental health, such as placing oneself in danger of sexual and/or violent attacks. In some cases, alcohol can increase violent acts by a person, or to a person. This is particularly evident when alcohol-fueled riots or large fights take place. These violent acts can cause serious and often long term damage to the mental health both perpetrators and victims, even resulting in Post-Traumatic Stress Disorder (PTSD).

Many serious psychiatric illnesses are either directly caused or exacerbated by alcohol, either used alone or together with illegal drugs such as methamphetamine (ice), cocaine or opioids. These include major depression, bipolar disorder and alcoholic/drug-induced psychosis. Luckily, if caught in time, many can be completely reversed by abstinence.

Many illegal drugs can also make anxiety worse. Cannabis for example, is very good at easing anxiety in the short term and in small quantities, but if you overuse it, it can make anxiety worse. Other drugs, such as cocaine, ice, amphetamine, opiates etc., are just bad for you in general, and addictive, and are not going to help your anxiety at all. If your drug use is becoming a problem, I strongly advise you seek medical and/or psychological help.

I personally find that the only way I can effectively use alcohol is NOT to use it at all. I don't drink to excess when I drink, but I drink habitually, and it makes me feel bad. I have an excellent technique for cutting down or giving up booze, which you can buy at Amazon[iii] (Breaking the Booze Habit, Amazon).

Not being able to exercise

Anxious people often use exercise to help cope with their anxiety.

Cardiovascular exercise in particular is very effective for anxiety (see more on this later). But of course, not all of us can exercise; even if we are used to regular exercise. Things such as illness, injury, travel, personal safety and so-on can impact on our ability to exercise---and anxiety and depression often make too stressed to exercise, or if you have a particular symptom, you may avoid exercise in case it triggers something. Quite often when I am anxious, I stop exercising---then I feel worse.

But if you are used to regular exercise, stopping has negative impacts on your body and your mind. Recently, I snapped my Anterior Cruciate Ligament (ACL) an important bit of the knee that helps stabilize the upper and lower parts of your leg. I'd always used exercise to cope with anxiety, mostly running and hiking---now all of a sudden, I could barely walk, let alone run. Even though I knew this was going to happen, and tried to prepare for it, the lack of exercise triggered an anxiety episode lasting some months, where I was convinced one spot after the other was cancer; as soon one was removed, I'd notice another, and the whole cycle would start again.

If you do not exercise, and you are able to (and most people can at least walk, or swim if you have joint issues) then you should consider starting. I'll talk about this later in the section on what to do, but lack of cardiovascular fitness is very bad for our bodies---and is implicated in many serious illnesses, such as heart disease, some cancers and even Alzheimer's. Those of us who suffer from health anxiety should, of all people, start doing some exercise.

You DO have a health condition

Funnily enough, many people with health anxiety say they become *less* anxious if they actually get a serious illness. It is almost as if the fear of getting the disease is worse than the actual disease. Most of us are strong people and are able to cope quite well with bad things that happen to us or our loved ones.

Nonetheless, being told that you have a health condition can cause extreme anxiety, particularly if it is life threatening. Even if the health condition is quite minor, we get anxious thinking that the doctor may have misdiagnosed it, or it could progress to something worse. The medication might also cause side effects!

For example, many medicines have quite severe side effects, sometimes worse than the actual illness. And we all know that medicine for anxiety (more on this later) also has side effects. I used to go on Zoloft and stop it as soon as I felt better. However, this chopping and changing made the side effects so bad this time, that I thought they were evidence of the dread disease that I was currently having an anxiety attack about!

Unhelpful Health Related Thoughts

We are not dual! Our minds (brains) and body are a system, and are connected in every possible way. What we think affects our body, and what we do to our body affects our mind. Other systems within the body, such as the ecosystem of our gut bacteria, can also influence our thinking.

For example, recent research has strongly linked chronic inflammation in the body with depression[iv]. What is chronic inflammation? We all know what acute inflammation is; if you get an infected injury for example, the skin around the wound gets red, and hot, and sometimes swollen. However, chronic inflammation is different, and can last for years. It can be the result of autoimmune disorders such as asthma or rheumatoid arthritis, other diseases such as ulcerative colitis or hepatitis, or even gum disease and sinusitis; and exposure to low levels of irritants such as industrial chemicals. Most pertinently, it can also result from stress and/or a poor diet; high quantities of junk food, soft drinks, low fiber foods and lack of fruit and vegetables.

Chronic inflammation can be detected by blood tests, but even if you do not go to the doctor, you can improve levels of inflammation by reducing overall stress levels, eating better (especially the Mediterranean diet of fresh vegetables, fruits, nuts, and oily fish), eating fewer inflammatory foods (fried foods, soft drink, red meat and junk food), doing regular exercise 2-3 days a week, mind-body practices like meditation and yoga, and breathing exercises (Ch5).

CHAPTER FOUR: HOW HEALTH ANXIETY IS MAINTAINED

Health anxiety is maintained by unhelpful health rules and assumptions, which are exacerbated by specific triggers. These lead to people wanting control, checking, and catastrophizing (see below) about their symptoms, misinterpreting information from the doctors and the media, assuming that they will not be able to deal with the problem if it is serious, and focusing only on the negative.

Control

One of the main contributors to health anxiety is the need for control. This is common to many of the anxiety disorders, most marked in OCD. People with health anxiety don't like uncertainty and the feeling of being out of control; they tend not to like surprises or not knowing what is going to happen. Conversely, having health anxiety is like feeling that no matter what we do, nothing is under control. Pema Chodron, a Buddhist nun and teacher calls this 'groundlessness' and says that we need to cultivate groundlessness, and to be comfortable with not feeling the 'ground' under our feet; because, of course, we are really in control over very little in our lives.

The main reason for this is FEAR! I have capitalized this, because it is so important. I rejected, argued and fought against this idea for years; mostly because I like to see myself as strong and independent. But if we really unpack what is behind our health anxiety (and any anxiety) it is fear---fear of death, fear of the unknown, fear of pain, fear of a million different things.

Now, fear is normal; people without fear are the odd ones out, but those of us with health anxiety have very sensitive fear antennae. Often, we've experienced situations, particularly in childhood, where we haven't had much control over our lives, and we've feared loss, abandonment and other difficult things. Many of us have experienced these in our own lives, which makes it worse.

What happens in childhood in particular, is that a person having experienced bad things, especially if they are unexpected, like a person dying suddenly or being sent off to boarding school, starts to crave security, and control over their life.

Now, much of life is beyond our, or anyone else's control, but we can do many things that can give us the feeling that we are, at least temporarily, in control. We can control our environment by keeping it clean and hygienic, we can control our bodies (to some extent) by being careful what we eat and by exercising, we can control our emotions by burying them so they don't come up and distress us, and we often try and control others, such as partners. But we **can't really control** any of this, which is why what we've buried often manifests in symptoms like health anxiety, anorexia or OCD.

With health anxiety, we try and control the chances of getting a serious illness by constant checking in case something is going to go wrong, or by visiting the doctor at the slightest symptom or, seemingly illogically, avoiding everything medical in the hope that it will just go away. Health anxiety and OCD are deeply connected, and many of us with health anxiety have some degree of OCD. Indeed, the same SSRIs are used for both conditions (see later).

There are effective means by which we can release our need for control, and it will likely make us happier people as well as less anxious. I will discuss these in the Solutions section, but just to note that one of the most effective means to release control is to practice some of the Buddhist and other meditation techniques

Catastrophising

I could write an entire book on catastrophising, which is a particular characteristic of health anxiety, often differentiating it from some other types of anxiety. Catastrophising means to take the worst possible interpretation of something; someone is late arriving, therefore they have died in a car crash; you find a weird spot, therefore it is stage 4 melanoma and you are going to die a horrible, painful death; you have palpitations, therefore it is an imminent heart attack. You get the picture!

One way that catastrophising 'works' with health anxiety is that every symptom is seen as a sign of a serious illness; no matter how severe the symptom or how long you have had it. You feel a sudden twinge of pain in your lower back, and immediately think it is the first sign of an advanced cancer; or you feel pain in your shoulder, and it's an imminent heart attack---never mind that you spent the previous day digging up the garden or doing an intense workout.

Catastrophising also means that the perceived illness is immediately viewed as serious, and most likely fatal. Even if your spot did turn out to be melanoma, most are found in the easily cured stage 0 or 1 melanoma (particularly as those with health anxiety tend to check their skin religiously). Catastrophising means that you think it is bound to be stage 4 nodular melanoma which has already spread, therefore you are doomed, to a long drawn-out, painful death. Media stories of such things do little to help; they try and publicise certain conditions, by using personal stories, but almost always, they end in death!

People who catastrophise tend to do this for other things than health, and about other people too; you may misinterpret someone's bad mood as meaning that they hate you, are immediately convinced you are going to be fired if you stuff up something, thinking your partner is having an affair if they are late coming home---a million other ways you misinterpret reality.

I am a terrible catastrophiser, sometimes to ridiculous extent. I went overseas a couple of years ago, and I tend to get petsitters who are all Luddites, no mobiles, no internet, no social media. Anyway, I wanted to contact my pet sitter to let her know what time I would be back, but she was not answering the phone. Instead of assuming she was out, I kept phoning from various airports, and constructed an elaborate scenario that she had died in my house, and my pets had eaten her. I have a very good imagination! Of course, she was fine, just out!

You can also misinterpret the information that your doctor tells you; although this is partly the fault of the doctors for not explaining better. For example, some blood work results change regularly (for example, thyroid stimulating hormone or cholesterol) and your results may be slightly abnormal one time, and within normal range the next. This particularly applies to blood tests which require fasting, as a lot of us don't really pay all that much attention to the instructions not to eat after a certain time, or conveniently forget that late night snack, or think that drinking (anything) doesn't count. Last time I had blood tests, my doctor said I was anemic, so I instantly panicked, conveniently forgetting that I had donated blood two weeks previously (and a week earlier than the recommended 12 week minimum---and I'd volunteered for a study and they'd taken 100ml of blood the day before), and my other doctor had told me years ago not to donate blood more than twice a year at most!

Catastrophising is characterized by certain common features: black and white thinking, lack of perspective, magical thinking, fear, ambiguity and lack of control. In brief, black and white thinking is 'either/or' thinking; either it is the worst possible outcome, or everything is wonderful. This ignores the concept that everything falls along a continuum, in about a billion shades of grey.

The lack of perspective is similar; it is very difficult to be rational when you are in full catastrophic flood. It is a bit like anxiety at 3am. I'm sure you all know what that feels like, you start ruminating over something you did, or didn't do, or are worried about or whatever, and the next thing, it is 5am, you haven't slept a wink, and whatever it is has been magnified into something huge. Usually, however, once you are awake and have had a couple of cups of coffee, and start thinking more rationally, the problem reverts to its actual, rather insignificant, reality.

I think that magical thinking is one of the major causes of catastrophising. Magical thinking is quite complex, but it means that if you think a certain way about something, you *think* that will either prevent it happening, make it happen or be prepared for when it does happen. Magical thinking is common in anxiety; we all have our major health fears and often avoid even speaking the name of the dread disease aloud in case it somehow causes us to have it. Magical thinking in catastrophising is almost the opposite: you think and emotionally live the worst possible outcome, so that IF it does happen, you will be prepared for it. But in reality, how often has the worst outcome actually happened, or even if it was bad, was it AS bad as you imagined? If you are constantly 'living' through the worst outcomes of something, then it is possible that you spend most of your life having horrible emotions, fears, griefs etc...all for nothing.

Fear goes without saying, so I won't go into further detail (it is covered in other sections). The lack of control and ambiguity are very similar; anxious people typically like to have control over their lives, and prefer as little ambiguity as possible. So, after I tripled my running distance in two weeks, and had a horrible trip running downhill in a trail run, and then, my lower back suddenly went with that horrible 'snap' and I couldn't walk for a week, I was not particularly ambiguous about the cause of my pain. But, if I have upper and middle back pain, which I frequently get from bad posture, which comes on slowly and characteristically on one side, then I almost always get paranoid that it *might* not be muscular but something horrible like lung cancer.

I speak of lack of control elsewhere, but it is really characteristic of anxiety. Us anxious people like to have control, pretty much over everything in our lives. Not knowing something is way worse than having the real facts! But we can never have complete, or even partial control over our lives! Meditation and mindfulness helps very well with this.

Checking

Checking is the WORST part of health anxiety (well, not really, but it seems that way sometimes). Constant checking is very similar to what people with OCD report, which is why health anxiety and OCD are often treated with the same medications. People with health anxiety report frequent:

- "Checking in the mirror for signs of asymmetry, areas of discolouration, or new moles or lumps

- Poking, palpating or pinching of the skin, breasts, stomach or other areas of the body
- Examination of bodily excretions (e.g., saliva, urine, feces) for signs of blood or infection
- Measuring parts of their body (e.g., using tape measure or calipers)
- Monitoring bodily processes (e.g., taking pulse, checking blood pressure)
- Weighing their body or bodily excretions
- Asking family members, friends, and health care providers about their symptoms
- Researching their symptoms on the internet or in medical texts
- Posting their symptoms on internet sites to obtain others opinions about their symptoms
- Requesting medical tests or evaluations, and second opinions" [i]

One problem with checking, apart from the stress it causes, is that the poking and prodding of the offending area often *causes* it to become swollen or inflamed, or to change colour. Moreover, it is sometimes very difficult to remember what the spot or lump looked or felt like *before* you noticed it, so that you may think it has changed, but it has stayed the same, or if it has changed, the change is normal. Just look at the skin of a very old person, who has spent most of their life in the sun, to see what you or might think are hundreds of suspicious lesions!

Checking can manifest very quickly. The other day, I noticed a change in one of my moles (which I monitor weekly). I instantly panicked, more so when the red spot (literally about ½ mm in size) fell off and began to bleed. I instantly diagnosed melanoma, although it looked like a scratch and scab. I started with my usual checking, but after picking at it over a day and making it look worse, I decided to put a Band-Aid on it, and leave it all weekend (figuring that if it were 'bad', it wouldn't kill me in two days) and if it were a scratch, it would heal by then. It was SO difficult not to check it! Still, on Monday, after a sleepless night, I sat on the loo, holding the toilet paper in my hand, when my cat jumped up and tried to bat it out of my hand! She missed---and scratched my thigh in the very same spot as the new lesion! I took off the Band-Aid and found it had healed---and remembered that the cat had scratched me there the previous week!

The psychologists call checking a safety or reassurance behavior; and it is encouraged by medical professionals, governments etc.; we are constantly told to check for signs and changes and symptoms, so that we can catch something early. Checking also gives us short term relief from our anxiety; we worry about something, so we check it (or go to the doctor to be reassured), which then gives us relief and control---in the short term. But it does not solve our problems in the long term, as we cannot know what might go wrong in six months, a year, or six years. We can't take our bodies to the 'mechanic' and say we need a guarantee that nothing is going to go wrong (though I did read today that there is a blood test that can tell us how much longer we might live)[ii]. To be honest, if you have health anxiety, do you *want to know* that you are going to develop cancer in ten years? Especially if it is a type that you can't prevent.

We need to build up our tolerance to uncertainty, and lack of control; strengthen the muscle of tolerance so as to speak. This is how many of the techniques described in Chapter 5 work, they expose you, like phobia treatments, to slowly increasing levels of what you are afraid of. If you constantly 'run away' from your fears, they get bigger and bigger and more terrifying.

This is a technique used by despotic governments and the like to reinforce fears. For example, in apartheid South Africa, the government deliberately kept the different cultural groups separate, because if you don't have any experience of other people, you don't know what they are really like. Demonising other races makes them as 'other', and easier to foment hate for them, out of fear. If you know that Mary or Mohamed or Lu Xing are just the same as you, with the same fears, loves, hates, and sorrows, then you are far less likely to want to be separate from them. Well, the same applies to fears, if you know that something is not as bad as you imagine (see catastrophising), then you are less likely to be terrified of it.

Of course, checking is not necessarily bad, and you *should* check certain health indicators at certain intervals. In the absence of any symptoms and risk factors, and say you live in a place like Australia, it is a very good idea to have a skin check at minimum once a year (more regularly if you have had skin cancer before, or you have risk factors such as fair skin and red hair). The same goes for certain health checks such as cholesterol, blood sugar, blood pressure, etc. The problem with checking is when it becomes too frequent or even 'obsessive'.

Some people are the total opposite, and never check (this too may reflect health anxiety, or avoidance behavior), but many with health anxiety don't just check their skin or breasts or other physical symptoms once every couple of months, but weekly, daily or multiple times a day. The checking may also involve asking others, taking multiple tests, browsing the internet, or going to the doctor too frequently---despite being reassured. I once browsed through at least 50 pages of pictures on the internet until I finally found one that (I thought) looked like what I had (an extremely rare and aggressive type of skin cancer---which turned out to be an infected splinter).

To start to cut down on checking, you need to identify a behavior that you want to modify, such as checking certain moles for changes. You also need to ask yourself whether this is doing any good, is it sensible to do it so often, and what advantages (or disadvantages) does it give to me?

Also, does the behavior cause you to act strangely, or hide things from other people? I wore socks for two months in the middle of the Australian summer, so people wouldn't see the terrible lesion on my ankle and <horrors> ask if I had had it checked out by a doctor (it was literally about 2mm in size). And I'd only bath in darkness, with a candle (I hope my housemate wasn't too confused by that!) Do you feel that you have to go elsewhere to check yourself; or that if you don't check yourself, then something terrible is going to happen? It is a genuine compulsion to check, and can be very distressing.

There are a number of ways to work on checking, one of which is to **postpone** the checking to a specific time or limited duration. So, instead of checking your skin every time you go to the toilet, you might say, I will only check my skin from 5pm to 5.30pm; or I will only check myself on a Monday morning at 7am. You might also say, I will only check myself for 30 minutes a day this week, 25 minutes a day for next week, 20 minutes the following week and so on. At the same time, you can diarise how much distress it causes you *not* to check yourself, and by slowly weaning yourself off checking, you can begin to reduce the number of checking times to a more manageable level.

There are other methods you can use to reduce checking, including keeping busy, distracting yourself, and even 'hiding' the object (mostly for skin lesions). I put a Band-Aid on myself, say on a Thursday, and say, I will only check this mole on Monday, because checking it over a weekend will not do me any good, and if it really looks changed, then I can make a doctor's appointment. You have to be strong though as it is incredibly difficult not to check! One thing to remember is that any emotion literally only lasts 90 seconds! It is easy to distract yourself for a minute and a half, and the more you work on delaying the checking, the easier it gets (it does, really).

Avoidance and safety behavior

Have you ever had something you had to do, that you put off for days and days? And the longer you put it off, the harder it was to do it? Some people put off difficult things for months, or even years!

Many of us with health anxiety practice avoidance behavior, for fear it will trigger an anxiety episode. These behaviors might be avoiding stories in the media about feared health conditions, visiting people who have been sick or even contacting people who have the disease that we most fear, not wanting to walk past or even look at signs for doctor's surgeries, hospitals, funeral homes, or cars with logos of medical testing laboratories (one of mine). Avoidance behavior can also include stereotypical OCD type behaviors, such as extreme fear of germs, handwashing, or using public toilets. And of course, what is one of the worst, avoiding phoning for test results---and being terrified in case your phone rings and it is the doctor!

Safety behaviors are a type of avoidance and can even include magical thinking. These could be things like carrying antiseptic hand sanitizer, wearing a face mask in flu season, or trying to hold your breath if you have to go to a doctors surgery or hospital. Some are superstitious safety behaviors, such as having to touch certain objects at specific times in case 'bad luck happens' or wearing certain clothes when you visit the doctor (clothes that you wore the previous time you went to the doctor and your test results were negative, for example). I do all of these!

False stories (real but not true)

Tara Brach has a saying, real but not true. What does she mean by this? Well, as she says, just think of an apple, biting into the crisp flesh and the lovely taste---now compare that to a biting into an actual apple. The real thing is nothing like the imagination, as good as it might be. So with your thoughts; they are real, they exist, but how do you know that they are true? What evidence do you have that your stories are true?

So, if you are prone to catastrophizing, you will tend to tell yourself stories; your mind goes round and round endlessly on the terrifying scenarios dreamed up by your brain. But how many times have your stories and scenarios come true? Be honest. Much as we'd like to believe (or not like) in foretelling the future (preferably the winning Lotto numbers), there is no scientific evidence for this, and people like James Randi put up US$1 million as a prize if anyone came and proved their paranormal activities (after 19 years, no-one ever claimed it)[iii]. Even if the worst possible (in your mind) scenario comes true, it will almost certainly bear no resemblance to your imagination.

The stories that we tell ourselves have a deeper truth to them too; they can reflect stories that were told to us, long before we could even remember. Are the stories telling you that you are stupid and worthless; that nothing good in life will ever last; that you are doomed to failure? Many of these are stories that we've either directly or indirectly heard from parents, teachers, priests and other figures of authority. Maybe they were well meaning and didn't want you to get big headed; maybe you just internalized the way that they dealt with things in life; maybe you were just born with your happiness meter set a bit lower than everyone else. Whatever the reason, if we can recognize these stories, we can stop them; we can say, yes, you are real, but you are not true.

Overthinking (over analyzing)

First, what do I mean by overthinking? Overthinking can mean either going over and over what happened in the past, like, did my boss think I was being weird when I said something; or as most health anxious people do, about the future, what does this symptom mean, am I going to die? It also means to go over problems until they get bigger and bigger and bigger. The more you go down the spiral of overthinking, the less rational you are about a problem, because you are now looking at it from the bottom of the well. As Einstein reportedly said, **'We can't solve problems by using the same kind of thinking we used when we created them'**.

Am I going too far to say that all people with health anxiety are over thinkers? Perhaps not. There are some people in life who seem miraculously able to NOT endlessly ruminate on stuff, who can just be in the moment without a second thought, who can make decisions without going through 500 hundred permutations, who can just pack up and go on a trip without sleepless nights wondering what might go wrong. Are there people like that? I suppose so, but they are completely alien to anyone with anxiety.

Those of us with health anxiety on the other hand are rabid over thinkers (maybe I shouldn't say that word, I used to be terrified of rabies as a child). We are however the type of people who on one hand are most drawn to meditate (to quiet our minds if nothing else) and on the other hand, find it incredibly difficult NOT to think.

Our brains are wonderful tools and they can do incredible things; and the same applies to our capacity to think. You would not be able to read this, nor me write it without thinking, but all too often, we elevate our thinking to the highest possible order, like some deity sitting on top of a mountain. Not every situation in our lives requires extensive analysis, or we'd be constantly exhausted. The problem is, many people with anxiety DO overthink almost everything. My oldest son for example, will go over and over and over the pros and cons of buying something, like a mobile phone or computer, and will keep phoning me asking for my advice (because I am a geek and love tech)! But even though I am also an anxious person, I am NOT anxious about things like that; for example, I have a large wardrobe of stuff that doesn't fit me and doesn't look good on me, because I am impatient and hate shopping and just randomly buy stuff without trying it on or because I am bored and want to go home. So I say to him, oh just buy the cheapest, or the one that looks the best, and he gets very annoyed with me!

Anxiety

Anxiety also triggers more anxiety! Because we have a symptom, or are feeling a bit off, we get anxious. The problem is, anxiety *causes* more symptoms, and can make existing symptoms worse, and make us think we have something terrible. Some symptoms resulting from anxiety (and the chemicals it releases) include[iv]:

- muscular tension, backache, knotted muscles, general achiness, headache, neck and shoulder pain, numbness and tingling, muscle twitches, burning skin, flushed face
- tiredness, exhaustion or sleepiness, lethargy, weakness, losing (or gaining) weight
- skipping, racing or pounding heart, palpitations, changes in breathing rate / breathlessness, chest pain or pressure (**don't ignore these symptoms though**)
- dizziness, light-headedness, blurred vision, confusion, feelings of unreality, brain fog, brain zaps.
- hyperventilation, feeling dizzy, sweating, shivering, night

　　　　sweats, hot flushes
- widening of the pupils, blurred vision, spots before the eyes, a sense that the light is too bright
- a dry mouth, nausea or an upset stomach, constipation, gas, stabbing/stitch like pain in abdomen…and more…

(source CCI, Module 3 & No More Panic Health Anxiety Forum, Anxiety Central Forum)

Her Diary:
Tonight, I thought my husband was acting weird. We had made plans to meet at a nice restaurant for dinner. I was shopping with my friends all day long, so I thought he was upset at the fact that I was a bit late, but he made no comment on it. Conversation wasn't flowing, so I suggested that we go somewhere quiet so we could talk. He agreed, but he didn't say much. I asked him what was wrong; He said, 'Nothing.' I asked him if it was my fault that he was upset. He said he wasn't upset, that it had nothing to do with me, and not to worry about it. On the way home, I told him that I loved him. He smiled slightly, and kept driving. I can't explain his behavior I don't know why he didn't say, 'I love you, too.' When we got home, I felt as if I had lost him completely, as if he wanted nothing to do with me anymore. He just sat there quietly, and watched TV. He continued to seem distant and absent. Finally, with silence all around us, I decided to go to bed. About 15 minutes later, he came to bed. But I still felt that he was distracted, and his thoughts were somewhere else. He fell asleep - I cried. I don't know what to do. I'm almost sure that his thoughts are with someone else. My life is a disaster.

His Diary
Motorcycle won't start…can't figure out why.

CHAPTER FIVE: HELPFUL THINGS TO DO

This section is all about things you can do to help your health anxiety. I have tried most of them, some of which work better (for me) than others. Others might find that different techniques work better---we are all different. I have separated these into two categories, long term and crisis interventions. Long term interventions can of course be used during a crisis, but crisis interventions are more practical when you are going through an episode of health (or other) anxiety. Both long term and crisis interventions do two basic things---change the way you think, and change the environment around you (this may include your own personal environment, such as your body!) Of course, some of the long term interventions can be used in a crisis and vice versa.

LONG TERM INTERVENTIONS

Counselling and Psychology

Firstly, counselling is *the* most common and possibly most effective method of dealing with anxiety. As with types of anxiety, and ways to combat it, there are hundreds, if not thousands of different types of counselling. I will give a brief overview what counselling is, what it entails and how effective it can be, then I will discuss a couple of the most effective (and common) counselling practices used for anxiety, Cognitive Behavioral Therapy (CBT), Exposure Therapy and Mindfulness Based Cognitive Therapy (the latter is also referenced in the section on Mindfulness, so this part will be relatively brief). Of note, no psychotherapy is a quick fix, and also, it can be quite expensive, especially if you do not have private medical insurance and/or live in a place without socialised medical system.

Cognitive Behavioral Therapy (CBT)

CBT[i] is the most commonly used type of psychotherapy for anxiety (and depression). It combines cognitive therapy and behavioral therapy, and teaches people to change their negative thinking patterns into more positive thoughts. Unlike some psychotherapies, CBT is aimed to treat people within a limited period of time, as it requires fewer sessions, thus can be cheaper. CBT is a tool[ii] that aims to teach people techniques to deal with stressful situations, identify ways to manage emotions, cope with non-mental illnesses, work alone or alongside drug-based treatments, and help almost anyone deal with difficult times.

There are certain things that you should do before embarking on a CBT journey; in brief, find a therapist, research the costs and any insurance cover and limitations, check the qualifications of the therapist and whether they are certified and licensed in your State or County. Of note, not every therapist and person will be a good match, even if the therapist is the best in the area. The therapy relationship is just that, a relationship, and not everyone gets along. It is generally fine to have a preliminary meeting with a potential therapist before committing to some sessions; almost like a job interview, where you can find out about their approach, the length of sessions, cost, your and their goals for your treatment, and how many therapy sessions you need. Also, be aware that popular therapists, like all medical specialists, can be booked up many months in advance. CBT also aims for the therapist and the 'patient' to work together, and 'homework' is given.

In CBT, there are usually a number of steps; identify the issues that are concerning you, increase awareness of your thoughts, beliefs and emotions about these ideas, identify and reshape any negative or inaccurate thinking. Usually in the initial session, your therapist will ask you a series of questions, about the issue you want to address, your life and your goals.

Note, CBT is not often portrayed accurately in movies, if at all. Most movies (at least ones that I have seen) tend to portray Freudian talk therapy (with the archetypal patient on a couch) or less common forms of therapy, but ones that look good on screen, including hypnosis, shock therapy etc. CBT is a bit boring to watch!

CBT is only really effective if you are prepared to work with your therapist and do your homework. You are expected to participate in your treatment, and this may include keeping diaries, doing certain exercises etc. Also, even though it is relatively short term (compared to some other types of therapy), you still need to have a rapport with your therapist. I have seen many therapists in my life, and at least 50% I would not visit twice. This has nothing to do with the therapist, it is just that you need to find one with a 'good fit'. For example, if you are a middle aged woman, with adult children and having anxiety issues related to getting older, then it may be (not necessarily) better to see a therapist in a similar demographic. When my second ex-husband and I were splitting up (due to domestic violence on his part, no wonder I have issues with anxiety), one newly graduated couples counsellor was little help when discussing aspects about disciplining young children.

Exposure Based Therapy

I include this one, because it is the most effective treatment of phobias, and some other anxiety disorders[iii]. In essence, it is a type of therapy aimed at helping people overcome their fears, particularly phobias. Some recent research indicates that this type of therapy can be extremely effective in helping people with anxiety, even extreme anxiety such as found in PTSD[iv].

There's a saying in neuroscience that 'neurons that fire together, wire together'. This means that the more you think/worry/obsess about something, the stronger the pathway this forms in the brain. It's a bit like a dog behind a fence; every day it runs up and down along the fence barking at passers-by and other dogs. Eventually, it wears a deep rut in the soil, compacting it down hard. Even if you try and replant the grass, it won't grow unless you dig up the area completely. Well, that is what happens with habitual thinking; if you spend a lot of your time worrying what might go wrong, you are setting up a figurative rut in your brain.

Well, exposure based therapy is the therapeutic version of digging up the compacted soil[2];

Exposure based therapy works in a number of ways, by habituation (reactions to feared objects lessen over time), extinction (exposure 'digs up' the rut), self-efficacy (exposure teaches that you *can* cope with the fear), and emotional processing (change of belief about the feared thing or situation).

There are a number of ways that exposure therapy is conducted, but the most common are graded exposure, systematic desensitisation and flooding. The first two are similar, and the process is to slowly expose the person to what they fear, beginning with mild exposure and leading to actually confronting it. So, for a person with a phobia about spiders, the therapist may start with something like talking about spiders or showing pictures of spiders. Then a spider might be placed at a distance in a room, and slowly, brought closer, until the person is actually touching or holding the spider. With health anxiety for example, a person who is terrified of certain disease may choose to visit a hospice, or even just read about experiences of people who have had the disease.

Flooding is a more extreme, but very effective method exposure therapy, which in its purest form, means forced and prolonged exposure to the feared thing. This is not always practical in real life, as where would you get a room full of snakes! I used it quite successfully to cure my fear of heights---by going bungy jumping. Even though I was terrified, I was more motivated by not appearing to be a coward in front of my peers, than heights. Obviously I was not phobic though! With regard to flying, I have pretty much cured my fear of flying (unless there is really bad turbulence) by systematic desensitization (flying a lot).

---

[2] Hallucinogenic drugs also seem to offer promise in this regard, and are discussed under Medication

Change Your Mindset

Nearly all counselling and psychology aims to disrupt (change) your 'negative' thinking patterns and replace them with 'better' ones. Now, firstly, it is NOT that easy to change your mindset, and the so-called positive thinking/ affirmation type stuff WILL NOT WORK. I have had endless arguments with people (who don't have anxiety) who say, 'it's just your mind, think positively and it will go away'! Drives me demented! Anxiety is not something that people CHOOSE to suffer from, it is HORRIBLE! OK, rant over, but there is a way you can change your mindset.

I have only recently started doing this, and there are two ways that I do it. First, I put phrases or mantras in places where I can see them regularly (see, Real But Not True). These are on my bathroom mirror, and also on silicone bracelets that I wear all the time. I might even get the phases tattooed on my wrist! I discuss this later, but the second way I do this is to **challenge my anxiety** with my own self-image.

What do I mean by this? Well, I have a certain opinions about myself (whether they are true or not) and these clash with the way I behave when I am anxious. So it sets up what the psychologists call cognitive dissonance, which is the mental discomfort that occurs when you hold contradicting thoughts, or your thoughts and behaviours do not mesh---you are walking someone else's talk!

So, this example is entirely my own of course; but I like to think of myself as a strong, independent, capable person, who has endured and overcome quite a lot in my life. When I am going through an anxiety attack, I don't see myself as strong or capable. I see myself as a terrified little girl, in constant dread that something awful is going to happen and that I won't be able to cope with it. I know that this is nonsense, but I need to actively challenge these thoughts by telling myself over and over that I AM strong and brave----even if the worst were to happen.

A related aspect of this, and I am not sure if this is a negative or positive aspect of my own character, but I also deeply respect people who are strong and independent and brave, and don't respect people who behave as I do when I am in the throes of anxiety. In fact, I rather irritate myself, and think that I am being 'weak'. After a while, I find that because of this cognitive dissonance, I find the annoyance with my behavior starts to chip away at the anxiety! I have shared this because it works for me. However, be careful about using this technique as it could backfire, by creating a negative self-image, and making things worse. But, if you find it works for you, go for it.

Medication

Often, if you are struggling to cope with anxiety, your GP is the first person from whom you seek help. GPs can be extremely compassionate and of great help with anxiety, but they commonly prescribe anti-depressant/ anti-anxiety medication to people presenting with anxiety. Anti-anxiety medications do work, but not for everyone, and they also can have some rather unpleasant side effects. Sometimes it is worth trying other methods *before* medication, and if they don't work, then perhaps using medication. Medication also takes some time to 'kick in' so you have to persevere.

The most common medication used in anxiety disorders, including health anxiety are SSRIs (selective serotonin reuptake inhibitors)[v] and to a lesser extent, serotonin-norepinephrine reuptake inhibitors (SNRIs). At times, benzodiazepines such as valium and Xanax are also used, but can have severe side effects, and are addictive. Many people also take 'natural' remedies for depression, including St John's Wort, but evidence for their efficacy is sparse.

SSRIs

As mentioned above, SSRIs are the commonest prescribed medication for anxiety disorders. There are a number of different types including Prozac/ Sarafem (fluoxetine), Celexa (citalopram), Zoloft (sertraline), Paxil/ Paxeva/ Brisdelle (paroxetine) and Lexapro (escitalopram). These are commonly prescribed in doses ranging from 25mg and up. As with many drugs, their efficacy diminishes with time, so doctors will often prescribe higher doses. They also can have some severe side effects, which are frequently worse when going off the drugs. It is therefore important to taper off with slowly reducing dosages, rather than just going cold turkey.

Side effects of SSRIs include, loss of libido, weight gain or loss, nausea, dizziness, drowsiness or insomnia, headaches, dry mouth, gastritis, vomiting and diarrhea. However, most of the side effects are of relatively short duration, and only for about the first 3 months of taking the drug. I have only taken Zoloft, and found that the side effects did not last longer than about 6 – 8 weeks. It is also difficult to separate a possible side effect from an effect of just feeling better. For example, I tend to put on weight with Zoloft, but am not sure if this is from the drug, or just because when I am extremely anxious, I cannot eat and lose a lot of weight (of course, then I think I am definitely dying, as you know, rapid weight loss is a symptom of many dread diseases).

I usually go back on Zoloft if I am in an anxiety crisis/spiral and I just cannot get out of it. I only take 25 - 50mg and usually for about 3 – 6 months, and then stop taking it by tapering (cutting the tablets into halves and then quarters) over about 4 weeks. It does affect my libido, but this does not last long, and I am single and post menopause, and don't have much of a libido anyway. Other rather weird side effects (at least for me) are constant stuffy nose/ sinus blockage, and increased bleeding, like from gums. I have never had any side effects that people report when going off the drug, but I don't take a high dosage.

I have no experience with SNRIs or benzodiazepines, but the side effects are similar to SSRIs. SSRIs are the 'safest' type of anti-anxiety drugs, even for breastfeeding mothers, but they may not work for everyone. I would recommend that anyone considering going on medication for anxiety consider doing this in concert with other methods, such as exercise, mindfulness and counseling.

Always consult your GP or specialist before taking any medication (even natural medicines).

'Natural' Medicines

Social media in particular is rife with sites espousing the benefits of 'natural' medication to treat every single condition under the sun, including anxiety. However the scientific evidence for the vast majority of these is lacking. Moreover, there are hardly any controls on the supplement industry, and between and within brands, the amount of the substance may differ dramatically, and be cut with other things. Natural medicines are chemicals (as is everything on earth) just like pharmaceutical drugs, no matter what website tells you otherwise. They can also interact with other medication, either natural or pharmaceutical (as can things like grapefruit!) No matter how flashy the language and claims, if a site is trying to sell you something, they are a commercial organisation with a vested interest. Anyone can call themselves a scientist, and even if real scientists, are not necessarily specialists in that particular field of chemistry (or even in the natural sciences). If it sounds too good to be true, it probably is.

Natural remedies used to treat anxiety include kava, passionfruit root, valerian, chamomile, St John's Wort, omega 3 fatty acids, various homeopathic remedies, acupuncture and meditation (discussed elsewhere). The majority of these, with the exception of kava, have little, if any, rigorous scientific evidence to back up the claims, and their efficacy may be as a result of the placebo effect[3].

The effect of kava is promising for the treatment of GAD, but trials were not statistically significant[vi]. Kava can have serious, even fatal side effects, if taken to excess, including liver damage, and it interacts with a great many common medications[vii]. It should never be taken by pregnant or breastfeeding women.

---

[3] The belief that something will cure the ailment, and the subsequent cure (brain body connection)

Whenever taking a natural remedy, be sure to discuss this with your doctor (if you are on any other medication) as there can be negative interactions between many substances (for example, grapefruit and beta blockers). Also, bear in mind that some natural remedies can also have side effects, similarly to pharmaceutical drugs. If you are taking SSRIs, be particularly careful, as some natural remedies, including St John's Wort, could potentially give rise to a serious condition called serotonin syndrome. The side effects of St John's Wort also include mild stomach upset, allergic skin reactions, tiredness, restlessness, anxiety, sexual or erectile dysfunction, dizziness, photosensitivity, vivid dreams, diarrhea, tingling, dry mouth, headache, and liver injury. I have taken this, and had no side effects, but like everything, the dose makes the poison[4].

CBD Oil

Recently, there have been some small studies (and lots of anecdotal evidence[viii]) showing that CBD oil can help with anxiety[ix]. CBD (or cannabidiol) is not the same as the 'active' ingredient in marijuana, i.e. THC. Much CBD oil is made from hemp and not from cannabis and will not make you high. It can, however, make you fail a drug test (if that is something you have at your employment, or on the roads in your country). In some countries, you can buy it anywhere, but in others, such as Australia, you need a doctor's prescription.

One way that CBD oil seems to help with anxiety is it is a natural anti-inflammatory. Inflammation is normal in response to injury or illness, but when it becomes chronic, it is linked with many conditions, including depression. CBD oil may even decrease activity in the amygdala, which we learned earlier, is linked to anxiety. Some people use CBD oil to treat anxiety that they get from excessive cannabis use!

There are hundreds of brands of CBD oil on the market, and due to the market being unregulated, many of them have widely differing

---

[4] All things can be poisonous if taken in excess, even water

concentration and quality of CBD. Some also have significant quantities of THC---so WILL make you high. Try and source quality CBD oil (Google for brands) that is made from hemp and not cannabis. Also, if you are in Australia, you can buy it online or overseas if you are travelling, but it will probably confiscated by Customs[x] (in Australia, it is a Schedule 4 drug that needs to be prescribed, but whether you can a) get a prescription or b) find a pharmacy that stocks it, is another story). It is also available in lotions, tablets and chocolate!

Despite the (mostly anecdotal) evidence that CBD oil helps with anxiety, this may just be from the placebo effect. But the placebo effect is extremely powerful, and people can even respond positively to placebos if *they know it is a placebo*[xi]! People respond powerfully to the suggestion that something they are taking (or have had done to them) will help their condition, even if it is completely inert sugar pill. For example, people with knee pain who have 'fake operations' where a small incision is made, but no surgery is actually done, show the same amount of improvement (or lack of improvement) than those who have actual operations[xii]. In other research, people with IBS have been handed a placebo, told that it is a placebo, yet they still get better.

As all of us with health anxiety well know, our minds can amplify existing pain and even create pain. So, whether CBD oil is a placebo or it actually works, is probably irrelevant. If you can get some, give it a try. It has few, if any, side effects, and won't make you high (though that may be a disadvantage to some people!)

Hallucinogenic Drugs

These have some promising applications in the treatment of anxiety, depression and PTSD. Mostly still illegal, various hallucinogenic substances have been found to rapidly ease symptoms, with few side effects lasting any longer than the drug 'high'. Promising hallucinogenics for anxiety include psilocybin (magic mushrooms), MDMA, ketamine, LSD, and ayahuasca. A single dose of psilocybin under controlled conditions significantly eased anxiety and depression in late stage cancer patients[xiii]. Moreover, despite some temporary side effects, mainly hallucinations, and nausea, the positive effect of the single dose on their symptoms lasted for months. These have been used to effectively treat very severe types of depression and anxiety, which is resistant to more standard treatments, and with very few side effects.

Apart from psilocybin, there have also been promising results from the other drugs mentioned above. Both SSRIs and hallucinogenics seem to work on serotonin. SSRIs block the uptake of serotonin by the brain---hence making it more available, but hallucinogenics seem to change how the different parts of the brain communicate with each other. It has been hypothesized that they rearrange the 'neurons that fire together' to new pathways, thus ploughing in the ruts created by constant worrying. Unfortunately, these substances are illegal in most countries, and if available are likely to be 'cut' with potentially harmful substances (and in non-controlled amounts). Hopefully in time, they will become more widely used in treating anxiety and other mental health disorders.

Exercise

I cannot emphasize more strongly how beneficial exercise is for overall health, and for anxiety, depression and stress. But I also cannot emphasize more strongly that you don't need to be *good* at exercise to reap its benefits. Indeed, many people who are terrible at sport are the ones who stick at it the longest, and if you wait long enough, you are bound to last longer than everyone else.

I have exercised all my life, despite a complete lack of ability. But I love exercise, particularly running and hiking as they have so many benefits. It is wonderful for remaining calm and easing anxiety, maintaining a normal weight, good for thinking and brain health---and for those of us with health anxiety, it is absolutely fantastic for your physical health. Exercise has been proven time and again to reduce your lifetime risk of diseases like heart disease, diabetes and cancer. What better reason to exercise?

Where exercise really comes into its own is how it helps with anxiety. Indeed, many researchers have found that exercise is **as effective** as pharmaceuticals for helping with anxiety (and depression). Even better, you don't have to go and run for an hour or do sprints or something, you can just go for a nice walk, preferably in a natural environment, and it is equally as effective.

So, why is exercise so beneficial? Well, one way is that it improves blood circulation and general fitness---and health! And blood circulation is not just important for physical health, it is also important for mental health.

But what if you hate exercise? The good thing about exercise is that you don't have to do a specific type of exercise. There are hundreds of types of exercise, and if you detest running, loathe swimming or despise team sports, you can always find *something* you like---or at very least, don't hate as much. Even better, if you are doing it voluntarily, you are not being pushed by anyone. When I run, people always comment that I look happy. I always answer, I AM happy, because I'm running for fun and not competition.

You can also modify the type of exercise you do according to the weather; if it is too cold or wet, you can exercise indoors; if it is too hot, you can do exercise like swimming, which cools you down; if it is too humid, you can join a gym where it is air-conditioned. If you like exercising alone, you can choose a sport like running or walking; if you like exercising in groups, you can join a running club, or netball team or any other sport, even something like rock climbing or dragon boat racing. The good thing about exercising when you are past school age, is that no-one cares how good you are; most people are just doing it for fun.

Of course, let's not forget that some people cannot exercise, due to illness or physical inability---but there are very few people who can do **no** exercise at all.

People with no legs have climbed Mt Everest, others with terminal cancer have completed the 4265km Pacific Crest Trail, and some have just run round the block, which is a huge achievement for some people. Recently I did a 12km hike with a lady who had done hardly any walking at all, and when we finished and she told me that she was 75 years old! I said that I know lots of people in their 30s who would complain about walking that far!

Faith

Faith in a higher power can be extremely effective in helping with health anxiety. For example, you might pray to God, Jesus or Allah, or you could call on Bodhisattva[5]. Because health anxiety is so intertwined with the fear of death, reading the holy works or other faith-based books can be very helpful. Additionally, the clergy of many faiths often attend the bedside of dying people, and because of their experience with death, speaking to a person such as a Priest, Imam or Rabbi, might help allay some of your fears.

Buddhism in particular has some very profound teachings on coming to terms with your own mortality. The Buddha taught that life is impermanent and all will eventually pass away, but even though our body will pass away, our spirit remains.

Even the most rational and even atheist scientists have profound views on living and dying; from an ecological perspective, we go back into the earth, and provide nourishment for other creatures; our genes live on in our children and other family members; and from a cosmological perspective, we are all star stuff, and eventually we return to the universe from whence we came.

---

[5] Note; I am not an expert on religions, please use your own religious beliefs in this regard

You want a physicist to speak at your funeral
You want the physicist to talk to your grieving family about the conservation of energy, so they will understand that your energy has not died. You want the physicist to remind your sobbing mother about the first law of thermodynamics; that no energy gets created in the universe, and none is destroyed. You want your mother to know that all your energy, every vibration, every Btu of heat, every wave of every particle that was her beloved child remains with her in this world. You want the physicist to tell your weeping father that amid energies of the cosmos, you gave as good as you got.
And at one point you'd hope that the physicist would step down from the pulpit and walk to your brokenhearted spouse there in the pew and tell him that all the photons that ever bounced off your face, all the particles whose paths were interrupted by your smile, by the touch of your hair, hundreds of trillions of particles, have raced off like children, their ways forever changed by you. And as your widow rocks in the arms of a loving family, may the physicist let her know that all the photons that bounced from you were gathered in the particle detectors that are her eyes, that those photons created within her constellations of electromagnetically charged neurons whose energy will go on forever.
And the physicist will remind the congregation of how much of all our energy is given off as heat. There may be a few fanning themselves with their programs as he says it. And he will tell them that the warmth that flowed through you in life is still here, still part of all that we are, even as we who mourn continue the heat of our own lives.
And you'll want the physicist to explain to those who loved you that they need not have faith; indeed, they should not have faith. Let them know that they can measure, that scientists have measured precisely the conservation of energy and found it accurate, verifiable and consistent across space and time. You can hope your family will examine the evidence and satisfy themselves that the science is sound and that they'll be comforted to know your energy's still around. According to the law of the conservation of energy, not a bit of you is gone; you're just less orderly. Amen. -**Aaron Freeman**.

Mindfulness (and Meditation)

These techniques are incredibly popular at the moment, and just about every media source has some information on how to become more mindful, how to use meditation for stress and anxiety, how to improve productivity by practicing mindfulness at work and so on. But how much of the hype is true, and how useful are meditation and mindfulness in helping health anxiety?

First, a bit about the practices (very brief, there's heaps of stuff online etc) then how they can be used with health anxiety, and finally, some sub-genres of mindfulness that are also useful, such as the 5 senses mindfulness exercise and forest bathing.

What are meditation and mindfulness?

Meditation is a technique or practice that originated in ancient times to concentrate the mind and achieve a mentally calm state. Most often associated with Buddhism, it has been practiced in most religions, including Christianity. It is said to help with anxiety, depression, stress and pain relief. There are many types of meditation, but they can be generalized into focused attention (concentrating on one thing such as the breath) and open monitoring (mindfulness).[xiv] Mindfulness can be as simple as paying attention to the present moment and not on the multiple distractions that abound. There are many techniques for both meditation and mindfulness, including some very useful apps such as Insight Timer.

Mindfulness and mediation practices can be used in two ways for health anxiety sufferers, everyday (daily) and crisis mindfulness. Practicing everyday mindfulness is a good way to develop the 'mindful muscle' so it is stronger when an episode (crisis) hits. There are multiple meditation and mindfulness techniques, books, videos and groups. If possible, it is good to find some classes nearby, where you can take part in some group meditation exercises. Often led by an experienced instructor, these offer valuable lessons on how to meditate. However, if you do not have access to such groups, there's an enormous amount of resources on the internet, via apps, or in books. Some people really get into meditation, and even go on long, often silent retreats. I couldn't possibly sit still for hours, let alone not talk! Like everything, practice makes perfect; even five minutes of meditation daily can benefit enormously.

I will briefly describe one type of everyday and crisis meditation, but of course, there are hundreds, if not thousands more. Like exercise, there's sure to be at least one type that can help.

Everyday mindfulness (forest bathing)

One type of mindfulness meditation which is easier to engage in (at least for me) is Shinrin-Yoku or Forest Bathing, where participants walk mindfully in natural environments, paying attention to all of their senses. Forest Bathing (or Shinrin-Yoku) originated in Japan, and means 'bathing' with all of our senses in forests or other natural environments. It's relatively recent but its roots go back millennia, to when we were in much closer connection to the cycles of the earth.

Nowadays everything in our society is too fast paced; sometimes all we do is hurry hurry hurry! Our anxiety is often triggered by modern day stresses: too much work, not enough work, kids, health, family, parents, partners and money. We also spend too much time on technology, in front of screens, indoors, in cars, and consuming. To help the stress and anxiety, we often turn to substances such alcohol or tobacco, social media or drugs, or we numb ourselves with what Tara Brach calls the spacesuit or onion self; layers of protection against difficult times. But this also numbs us from our environment, and stops us connecting with our senses, and nature.

One method to help ease some stresses, making them less likely to trigger anxiety episodes, is to mindfully reconnect with nature. We've an affinity for nature because we're part of nature, and grounding ourselves by touching the soil, the trees and the soil helps promote self-healing by boosting immune function, reducing inflammation and free radicals. We sleep better, are less stressed and have less anxiety and depression after touching the earth.

Forest Bathing has physical, mental and spiritual benefits: it can reduce blood pressure, boost natural immunity, reduce stress, anxiety and depression, aid concentration and foster a deeper connection to the natural environment and to the earth herself. For example, researchers in Japan sent two groups, either to either a city or forest site, and at each site, they had to sit for 15 minutes, then walk around the site for 15 minutes. The ones who went to the forest had decreased pulse rates and levels of cortisol (a stress hormone). Other studies show that forest bathing helps decrease blood pressure, glucose levels and stress markers. This doesn't apply to city 'bathers', for some, stress markers increased.

A study of nearly 500 people spending two of four days in nature, scores on anger, boredom, depression and stress on the forest days were much lower than the non-forest days, and the benefits lasted as long as 30 days afterwards. Of another 168 people who spent time walking in the forest or an urban setting, the forest group had lower levels of depression, anxiety, anger and fatigue. Moreover, these positive effects lasted longer than just the time spent in nature; and that doing these activities regularly can help maintain better physical, psychological and spiritual health.

Forest bathing can be truly beneficial. Perhaps you do not have the time to do it every day (it can take a couple of hours, even for a short distance) but you can do what is known as the 'sacred pause'. Before doing something, perhaps on your walk from your car to work, or before doing some of your normal busy work, stop. For even as short as 20 seconds, just look closely at something. This might be new leaves on a plant, or a rock, or a tiny spider. One Buddhist monk for instance, was asked why he meditated. His answer was, so I remember to look at the tiny purple flowers on the side of the road when I walk into town.

Basic Forest Bathing

- In a natural environment (can be a city park, but ideally somewhere with few or no people and where you can walk about 500m to 1km), spend a couple of minutes in silence, paying attention to the breath, perhaps doing a quick body scan

- Walk a little way along the path paying attention to the feeling of walking, the air moving past, the sounds around you, the sights and smells

- Now stop at anything that takes your fancy and spend a few minutes concentrating closely at what you can see; look at the tiniest details, for example, leaves, insects, moss or lichen on a tree trunk. How much more do you notice by doing this?

- Walk a bit further, then stop and feel different textures; leaves, rocks, bark or soil (careful of thorns etc.); touch with your palms then your fingertips, then press harder and see what difference it makes.

- Now walk on, paying attention to the sense of proprioception, or movement through the landscape. Feel how your body moves, and notice the movement all around you, the leaves of the trees, perhaps birds or small animals. Feel how your weight moves as you shift from one foot to another.

- Now find something you can crush, like a leaf (make sure it is not poison ivy or nettles), and smell it; smell some fresh earth or leaf mould. What differences do you notice? Do some plants smell different than others, and why might this be so?

- Walk to somewhere that has good (natural) sounds. Cup your hands behind your ears and turn toward any sound that catches your fancy. Note how amplified this makes sounds. Do sounds have emotions, do they change, do they stop?

RAIN

RAIN stands for Recognise, Allow, Investigate, and Nurture, and is a type of mindfulness invented by Tara Brach and other Buddhist teachers to help work with difficult emotions[xv]. People can do RAIN in any situation, and I have found it invaluable when feeling very anxious. It allows you to direct your attention at something other than the anxiety, and to clarify the real situation. It also, with time, helps you to overcome the unconscious habits that you use in your everyday life, including the desire to control things around you. The steps of RAIN are:

- **RECOGNISE** *the emotion/ what is happening.* If you suddenly feel anxious, or it has been building up for a while, take the time to recognise what you are feeling, both the mental and physical sensations. For example, you may suddenly feel dread or impending doom (common in anxiety), together with the physical sensations of shortness of breath, tightness in the chest or a clenched jaw (different in different people). Ask yourself, what am I feeling, what is happening inside of me right now? Look at your reaction with what Buddhists call a 'beginners mind', as if it is the first time that you have ever experienced these sensations.

- **ALLOW** *it to be, just as it is.* Don't try and change things. We don't like the emotions and sensations that accompany anxiety, so we immediately try and change things, by self-medicating, hurrying, doing other things or suppressing the feelings. Instead, just allow the emotions to wash over your body, as horrible as they are. We spend too much of our time trying to get rid of 'negative' emotions, but suppressing things just buries them, so they fester and rot, and come back to haunt us when we are least expecting them (see The Felt Sense Prayer below).

    Have you ever had a really good deep tissue massage from a physiotherapist? You know the feeling, when the physio digs his or her fingers deep into a knot of tension and pain? How at first it is absolutely agonising, and then it slowly goes away so all you feel is relief? That is what allowing (or consenting) difficult emotions can do; it is horrible and agonising at first, then the pain just goes. You feel exhausted afterwards, but refreshed.

Tara Brach says that you don't have to do all the steps of RAIN, and often the first two suffice, especially if it is just a sudden twinge of anxiety pain. But if you are going through a more intense experience, like a long-term bout of anxiety, a divorce, difficulties at work, financial problems, whatever; then it is worthwhile to do the last two parts of RAIN, Investigate and Nurture.

- **INVESTIGATE** *with kindness.* Firstly, investigate does not mean **analyse**! Anxious people are inclined to over-analyse and over-think everything, going over and over the different possible causes of the problem. Instead, Investigate means to ask things like 'what most wants attention', 'what am I believing', 'how does this emotion feel in my body' and 'what am I afraid to feel'? If you have spent your whole life avoiding or judging your own difficult emotions, as I have, then this can be incredibly difficult---but incredibly rewarding. This is why Tara calls it Investigate---with KINDNESS. As she says, if your child comes home from school crying, you first offer kind and gentle attention, you don't sit them down for an inquisition on what happened (well, hopefully you don't). The question, 'what am I too afraid to feel', is incredibly powerful.

- **NURTURE (or NON-IDENTIFICATION)**. First, to Nurture the self (putting your hand on your heart works really well), and to feel compassion for yourself. Anxiety often has its roots in childhood, and the anxious self can be a reflection of the terrified child who may not have had all their needs met, may have been abandoned, bullied or even abused. Nurturing your inner child helps them understand and grow. Non-Identification means that you have recognized, allowed and investigated the fear, but that you don't identify with it, it is THE fear, and not YOUR fear. Everyone feels fear, and we recognise that, and let it be.

The Felt Sense Prayer (unknown author)
I am the pain in your head, the knot in your stomach, the unspoken grief in your smile.
I am your high blood sugar, your elevated blood pressure, your fear of challenge, your lack of trust.
I am your hot flashes, your cold hands and feet, your agitation and your fatigue.
I am your shortness of breath, your fragile low back, the cramp in your neck, the despair in your sigh.
I am the pressure on your heart, the pain down your arm, your bloated abdomen, your constant hunger.
I am where you hurt, the fear that persists, your sadness of dreams unfulfilled.
I am your symptoms, the causes of your concern, the signs of imbalance, your condition of dis-ease.

You tend to disown me, suppress me, ignore me, inflate me, coddle me, condemn me.
I am not coming forth for myself as I am not separate from all that is you.
I come to garner your attention, to enjoin your embrace so I can reveal my secrets.
I have only your best interests at heart as I seek health and wholeness by simply announcing myself.

You usually want me to go away immediately, to disappear, to sleek back into obscurity.
You mostly are irritated or frightened and many times shocked by my arrival.
From this stance you medicate in order to eradicate me.
Ignoring me, not exploring me, is your preferred response.
More times than not I am only the most recent notes of a long symphony, the most evident branches of roots that have been challenged for seasons.

So I implore you, I am a messenger with good news, as disturbing as I can be at times.
I am wanting to guide you back to those tender places in yourself,
the place where you can hold yourself with compassion and honesty.
If you look beyond my appearance you may find that I am a voice from your soul.
Calling to you from places deep within that seek your conscious alignment.

I may ask you to alter your diet, get more sleep, exercise regularly, breathe more consciously.

I might encourage you to see a vaster reality and worry less about the day to day fluctuations of life.
I may ask you to explore the bonds and the wounds of your relationships.
I may remind you to be more generous and expansive or to attend to protecting your heart from insult.
I might have you laugh more, spend more time in nature, eat when you are hungry and less when pained or bored, spend time every day, if only for a few minutes, being still.

Wherever I lead you, my hope is that you will realize that success will not be measured by my eradication, but by the shift in the internal landscape from which I emerge.

I am your friend, not your enemy. I have no desire to bring pain and suffering into your life.
I am simply tugging at your sleeve, too long immune to gentle nudges.
I desire for you to allow me to speak to you in a way that enlivens your higher instincts for self-care.
My charge is to energize you to listen to me with the sensitive ear and heart of a mother attending to her precious baby.

You are a being so vast, so complex, with amazing capacities for self-regulation and healing.
Let me be one of the harbingers that lead you to the mysterious core of your being where insight and wisdom are naturally available when called upon with a sincere heart.

RAIN is not something that you do once, and all of a sudden, all your anxiety disappears. Unfortunately life doesn't work like that. There are no quick fixes. You need to do many rounds of this to see the positive impacts; but as with all major changes, it has lifelong benefits.

Yoga

Yoga can benefit anxiety in a number of ways, by exercising the body, releasing stiff muscles (a major cause of anxiety induced pain), and by breathing and mindfulness practices. We've discussed exercise earlier and will discuss breathing later, so will briefly talk about releasing stiff muscles and the yoga version of mindfulness. The breathing aspect of yoga, which is actually the core philosophy of yoga, is brilliant at helping anxiety, so that is why it has its own section.

Many of us with health anxiety have pain, particularly in areas such as the shoulders and lower back. This pain can of course, be from more sinister causes, but in the vast majority of cases, is from anxiety, poor posture, ageing and muscle strain[xvi]. Anxious people are often highly stressed, and their muscles can get into horrible 'knots' which can be extremely painful. These can be released by trigger point therapy, massage, and stretching. Yoga (and similar practices such as Pilates), if done correctly, can release a lot of tense muscles. It is also good for strength, balance and posture. For example, strengthening the abdominal muscles can help significantly with lower back pain.

One of the biggest benefits of yoga is the mindfulness aspect. Most yoga practices include at least 10 minutes of savasana (the rather ominously named, for those with health anxiety, corpse pose). A good yoga studio will teach you how to do savasana, particularly the very useful progressive relaxation. But yoga, if practiced correctly, teaches mindfulness throughout the whole 'class' (of course, you can do yoga without a class, but it is very useful to attend one if you are a beginner). The process of holding a stretch, moving smoothly to another, and focusing on your breathing whilst doing so, is an active mindfulness exercise. You have to pay close attention to your body, the postures, and your breath…and doing this means that you are not spending your time obsessing over your health.

I am not going to go into any great details about yoga, as there are many different types of yoga, which are suitable for all types of people, ranging from the rather intense 'power' or astanga yoga, to hatha and vinyasa yoga, and even chair yoga for those less mobile. If you live near any sort of town or city, there is bound to be at least one yoga class (they are often held in gyms too). But if you live more remotely, there are tens of thousands of websites, apps and the like.

One warning though, do be careful with yoga, as if you overstretch or do too much, it can also injure you. Find a good teacher (even online) and pay attention to what they say. This is probably more of an issue with people who know a bit about yoga, and who are quite flexible. My aunt, a yoga teacher, once told me, 'Heather, yoga is not a competitive sport!'

Bene Gesserit Litany Against Fear
I must not fear.
Fear is the mind-killer.
Fear is the little-death that brings total obliteration.
I will face my fear.
I will permit it to pass over me and through me.
And when it has gone past I will turn the inner eye to see its path.
Where the fear has gone there will be nothing. Only I will remain."
Frank Herbert, Dune.

Death Cafes

What on earth is a death café[xvii]? Well, it is an event where people get together over tea, coffee and cake and discuss death! The aim of death cafes are to 'increase awareness of death with a view to helping people make the most of the (finite) lives'[xviii]. Death cafes started in the UK in 2011, and now there are thousands of death cafes around the world, and participation is free. They are facilitated by psychologists, ministers of religion, or just interested people.

I attended a death café held at the Anglican Church of my local town (it was secular however). Despite the horror expressed by friends and family (who perhaps would benefit by attending a death café), I found it a very enlightening and supportive space. We sat in a large group, and each person expressed a reason why they had come, and whether they were afraid of dying. To my surprise, I was one of the only people who said they *were* afraid of death. Most of the attendees said they were not afraid of dying (admittedly, they were generally older than me, even though I am in my mid 50s).

Death cafes are beneficial for those suffering from health anxiety (which is, essentially, fear of death) because they discuss death, and people's experience of death, in a way that makes it seem normal (which it is). I found some of the stories told by people of accompanying their loved ones in their final time, extremely moving and beautiful. Death cafes are not grief counselling sessions, they serve to normalize death, as part of life.

Volunteering

One way to help with our own problems and anxiety is volunteering. You can volunteer to do almost anything, either officially through an organization such as a church or charity, or just by asking people if you can help them. Of course, you can help any people, but a really beneficial way to do this for health anxiety would be to volunteer in a hospice or aged care home, where there are people who are dying, either of disease or old age. This is related to death cafes, and desensitization, as mostly we are not exposed to the dying, and we've no way of confronting our fears, except by what we read (or avoid reading) in the media. I haven't personally done this because a) I am too scared, and b) I would rather do volunteering that doesn't involve people as I am an introvert.

But any volunteering can help with health anxiety, because it takes us away from our obsessive thinking about our health and into doing stuff for other people or the environment. Many anxious people can be quite isolated, even if just in our heads, and if we can force ourselves out of this, then it can help break the anxiety cycle. Of course, any social or other activity can do this too, but volunteering is sort of special. Humans generally feel good about being altruistic, and then the positive endorphins help us feel better. Also, if we help others, especially if they *actually have* the diseases we fear, then we can learn from their experience and very often, the dignity and strength with which they deal with their condition.

Of course, volunteering in a cancer ward or hospice is basically akin to the phobia-busting technique of flooding and may trigger panic attacks or similar in those of us with health anxiety, so do be careful. If you feel that you can do it though, it can be a very worthwhile exercise, and really help others. If you feel you cannot do it, there's always opportunities to help others or the environment, even if you just help your neighbor put out her garbage, or an elderly person to cross the road.

Talks and Podcasts

There are a number of very useful talks and podcasts that you can listen to online, or download on to your own device to listen offline in your own time. I download my favourite podcasts on to my mobile phone and listen to these on my drive to work. This benefits me in the long term but is also remarkably useful for distressing, say, if you are stuck in a traffic jam! Also, not listening to the news is distressing in itself. Of course, there are thousands and thousands of good podcasts, so I am just going to share a couple that I find really useful. Like exercise, it is specific to you, and you may not find the same speakers as inspirational, or I may hate one that you love---but you are bound to find at least one that you like.

Tara Brach

Tara Brach[xix] is far and away my favourite podcasting speaker. Her talks are about 60 minutes long and are completely free (though you can donate if you wish). Tara is an American psychotherapist, writer, teacher and Buddhist. She has a PhD in Clinical Psychology and has also completed a 5 year Buddhist teacher training course. Her talks cover all sorts of subjects, but I find the most useful are those on fear. I download talks from her website and listen to them on my drive to work every day. I can truly say that Tara is the most influential person, who I have never met, in my life, and only wish that I had heard her talk decades ago! I mention her work again in the Crisis Intervention Technique section, as well as in RAIN.

Byron Katie[xx]

Byron Katie has used her own experience with depression to come up with a technique to end suffering called 'The Work'. The fundamental principle of her work is that you should not believe your thoughts. Instead of getting depressed about why the world around her was not as she thought it should be, she chose to change her thinking and question her thoughts and meet reality as it is. I personally know so many people who suffer because they think that life *should* be a certain way, and get depressed or anxious when it is not. This equally applies to health---as I discussed in the beginning, what is health anyway? If I think health *should be* the complete absence of any symptoms, then whenever I get a symptom, which is inevitable with age, I will get anxious. Do look into her work, it is excellent, and also relevant for anxiety. Byron Katie's resources are freely available on her website.

The Anxiety Guy[xxi]

The Anxiety Guy is Dennis Simsek, a former professional tennis player, and expert on anxiety, including health anxiety. Many people find his podcast really helpful, as he discusses his own experience with anxiety and the techniques he uses to work through this.

CRISIS INTERVENTION TECHNIQUES

Breathing and mindfulness techniques

There are some excellent breathing techniques that really help with all sorts of anxiety. Breathing techniques work because when you are stressed and anxious, your heart beat and blood pressure increase, as does your breathing rate. Too fast breathing can lead to hyperventilation, which has as number of unpleasant symptoms such as dizziness, fatigue, choking sensation, tingling in the extremities, palpitations, shaking and chest pain! If that doesn't send us straight to the emergency room, then it could also bring on a panic attack.

In what was probably one of the most embarrassing episodes of my life, I was being interviewed for a position at a very upmarket game reserve in Africa (like, where all the celebrities go). The interview process lasted a week, and they wanted to see how we coped with the environment. Unfortunately, I developed a huge crush on one of the rangers. I was in such a hyped up state, I wasn't eating, just in a daze of youthful lust, when I started hyperventilating, and when my hands and feet started tingling and I got dizzy, I convinced myself that I had been bitten by a snake or scorpion. I panicked so much that I persuaded the manager to take me to the nearest doctor, at least an hour's drive away, who gave me a tranquiliser (diazepam) and told me to breathe into a paper bag. Suffice it to say I recovered, they sent me home the next day and I didn't get the job and nor did I get the game ranger.

I wish I had known about deep breathing back in 1982. Anyway, when you start to pay attention to your breath, and breathe deeply, this helps slow the heartbeat, reduce blood pressure and lower breathing rates. It also has beneficial effects on blood chemicals and stress hormones.

There are a number of breathing exercises that can help anxiety; I will detail three, belly breathing, 4-7-8 breathing and pranayama (or Wim Hof breathing[xxii]). I find the second of these incredibly effective for anxiety, as well as helping to go back to sleep in the middle of the night.

Counting 5, 4, 3, 2, 1 Technique

One really effective technique is what I call the Counting 5, 4, 3, 2, 1 Senses Technique). This is similar to forest bathing, and a technique I often use as a preliminary exercise to get people to get more in touch with their senses. It is really useful when you are in the throes of an anxiety attack, and your mind is obsessing about some illness. This is a remarkably effective technique and can be repeated as often as you wish.

This technique is really simple; for each sense, do it for as long or as short as you like and pay attention only to each object and nothing else
- LOOK at 5 different objects,
- LISTEN to 4 different sounds,
- TOUCH 3 different textures,
- SMELL 2 different scents, and
- TASTE 1 different taste.

Belly breathing:

Sit comfortably and relax. Place one hand on your chest near the heart, and one on the belly
1. Stretch out gently and then sigh out a breath through your mouth; and as you do that, relax your neck and shoulders and all the tense muscles around that area as you exhale. Don't push all the breath out, it is meant to be gentle.
2. Count to 3 or 4 without breathing, but ensure you relax
3. Inhale slowly through your nose, and as you do so, push your stomach out in an almost exaggerated manner. Feel it move under your hand. Inhale as deep as you can just by using the belly, if it starts moving into the upper body, stop.
4. Pause again, this time for longer than 3 seconds, but not so you feel stressed or breathless. Remember that you are breathing deeper than your normal fast shallow breaths.
5. Exhale through your mouth by using your belly to push the air out as much as possible.
6. Pause for a few seconds.
7. Repeat until you feel more relaxed

4-7-8 breathing

I find this exercise wonderful for stress relief. I first heard about it on the internet (where else) where it was being touted as a method to go back to sleep if you wake in the middle of the night. This is indeed true, but it is also wonderful for calming anxiety, or just prior to a meditation session.

1. Sit or lie down in a comfortable position. Begin as for the belly breathing exercise, with one hand on your chest and one on your belly.
2. Take a deep breath from the belly to the (slow) count of 4.
3. Hold your breath and count to 7.
4. Breathe out completely, from the belly, to the count of 8. Try and get all the air out of your body.
5. Repeat until you feel calm (for around a minute, or 5-10 times).

Pranayama/ Wim Hof breathing

Pranayama is a yoga breathing technique---in fact, it is the descriptive term for a number of yoga breathing exercises. I am not going to go into great detail about pranayama, as there are some great resources on the internet; but I also suggest that you do a few sessions with a qualified instructor, as some of the techniques are quite difficult. This one is an adapted pranayama devised by Wim Hof (or the Iceman)[xxiii], a Dutch guy who has about 21 world records for cold exposure, for doing stuff like sitting in ice baths for hours or climbing Mt Everest in shorts. This exercise takes a bit of practice, but is quite easy once you know how, and is remarkably relaxing. This technique has been scientifically tested to have multiple benefits, even physical health benefits[xxiv].

1. This technique is ideally done before eating in the morning, or just before you got to be. Sit in a comfortable position where you can expand your lungs freely. I find that half lying, as on a chaise longue with my head and torso against pillows, is the most effective way of doing this.
2. Take 10 or so deep breaths with a small pause at the end of each inhale and exhale.
3. Now, inhale through your nose, and then exhale in a short sharp burst as if you are blowing up a balloon. You do not have to exhale all the air in your lungs, and try to make the exhale shorter than the inhale.
4. Use your belly and solar plexus to push the air out. You may

notice tingling or dizziness. This is normal. Do this about 30 times.
5. After 30 breaths, draw in a deep breath and fill the lungs to their maximum, then let the air out and hold your breath as long as you can (until you need to gasp). If you time yourself, you will notice that you can hold your breath a long time like this (my record is 3.5 minutes).
6. Take a deep breath in, and hold your breath again for about 10 seconds. This is round 1.
7. Repeat two or three times.
8. Wim Hof recommends a cold shower afterwards (which I can only do in Summer).
9. You will feel really relaxed, and if you want to meditate after, you will find that you can sink much deeper into a meditative state without much effort.

What evidence do you have?

This is THE technique I find the most useful when I am in the middle of an acute anxiety episode. What it means is that you need to find rational **evidence** for your stories that you are telling yourself. I'll describe the technique then show how it is used with a (true) scenario.

To use this technique, you can write things down, or just do them mentally. Often writing things down helps clarify them in your mind, but if you are going through a really severe episode, it may trigger more anxious thoughts. The CCI worksheets[xxv] have a useful table that you can print out and write down your own thoughts. Basically, what you do is write (or say to yourself), '**what is the factual evidence for this thought**?' and '**what is the factual evidence against this thought**?' You can also write down things like how you are feeling, rate the intensity of your feelings and the physical sensations that you are feeling. In addition, you can work through exercises where you write how it would affect you if the worst were to happen, any other explanations for your symptoms, what is the most likely explanation and what you can do to cope with the situation in the present moment.

I tend just to stop at looking at the factual evidence FOR and AGAINST, but it is worthwhile to do the entire exercise. As an example of how I use the technique is, last year I was having a major health anxiety episode about a mole that I thought was melanoma. Now I get my skin checked regularly, and this one, though large, never really bothered any doctors. One day, I noticed that it seemed to have a microscopic lump on it---and I instantly panicked, thinking it had turned to nodular melanoma (a particularly aggressive type). So off I rushed to the skin specialist, who looked at it and said, had I noticed any changes? Well, on one hand, I wanted it checked out, and on the other, I was too terrified to say anything.

He then looked at again, and said that it had little grey filaments in it, which in 99% of cases are benign but can sometimes be cancer. Well, apart from his lack of tact, this instantly freaked me out so I demanded he remove it. I could only get an appointment in a fortnight and in the meantime had to go to a conference in another city; where I was completely useless, as I was in a constant state of dread. All I can say about my anxiety is that it's great for losing weight, as I cannot eat when I am in the throes of an attack.

On the way back, I noticed that I had swollen glands on one side of my neck. Oh my god, I thought, it has spread already. I constantly checked and poked and prodded it, and finally got it removed, where I was in a state of utter terror, which the nurse mistook for me being anxious about the operation. I am not in the slightest anxious about *that* as I have a very high pain threshold. Anyway, she said they'd ring if they found something. I figured it would be soon if it was cancerous, so I waited, and waited and waited---dreading the telephone ringing. I took it everywhere, and was more terrified of getting a missed call from the doctor's surgery than the actual call---which never came. Eventually, after a week, I *emailed* the doctor as I was too scared to phone. I was told, oh its fine, come back in a year! Oh, and the swollen glands? A tooth abscess!

I used the 'what evidence' technique to calm myself down.

1. The doctor wasn't particularly worried and had only removed it because I insisted;
2. he must see thousands of cancers every year (I live in Australia!);
3. no-one had rung me;
4. it could have been from something else, I vaguely remembered scratching myself there;
5. the lump hadn't grown; and
6. if I check my skin regularly, surely I would find something before it was too late.

So, rationally speaking, I had very little, if any, evidence that it was cancerous, and if it was, it was highly likely that I had caught it in time.

Real but not true

A related technique which can be used as part of the evidence exercise is the quote, 'real but not true'. I find this so useful that I even have silicone bracelet with these words. I first heard of this phrase from my favourite podcaster, Tara Brach[xxvi], a wonderfully wise meditation teacher, psychotherapist and Buddhist. She says to imagine an apple; if you have a really good imagination, you can almost see the shiny skin, the stalk, and the crisp flesh of the apple, and imagine the sweet taste as you bite into it. But no matter how good your imagination, your thoughts are not the actual apple. Your thoughts are REAL (they exist) but they are not TRUE (they are not the apple).

This technique works very well with health anxiety and catastrophising. If you are in an anxious thought spiral, thinking of increasingly dire consequences of your health problem, just say to yourself, 'real but not true'. Yes, all your horrible thoughts are real, they exist in your head, but are they true? How much do they reflect reality? The other day, I let my cat out, then later, in the shower after my morning run, I realised that I hadn't seen her since 5am, and started imagining that she had been run over, and suddenly descended into an anxious thought pattern about what would happen if I couldn't find her, or I found her limp body on the side of the road. I deliberately looked at my bracelet, and said, 'real but not true'. As I opened the door, she was there, waiting for food!

These two techniques can be effectively used to calm yourself down when things seem bleak and you are lost in imaginary dread. They may not make you 100% not anxious (are we ever 100% not anxious), but it can be enough to make you feel well enough to do another technique, such as exercise or meditation

Tapping (Emotional Freedom Technique)

The last time I was going through an anxiety episode, I went to see a psychologist, and he told me of this technique. To be honest, I dismissed it as pseudoscientific nonsense---until I tried it. It works very well in crisis situations, such as waiting to hear test results in the doctor's surgery, or taking off in aeroplanes (I hate take-off!) I'm not sure how it works as it is, indeed, based on some extremely diverse and not particularly scientific ideas, such as acupuncture, chi and Neuro-Linguistic Programming[6]. But before we dismiss it outright, just remember that the Chinese had medicine long before Westerners did; and even if it only works through the placebo effect (belief in the efficacy of a treatment), it still works, and especially in the treatment of some phobias[xxvii].

How it works is that there are certain points[xxviii] on the head and upper body that are considered meridian points or areas where we can work on 'energy disruptions'; the top of the head (TOH), inner corner of the eyebrow (EB), side of the eye (SE), under the eye (UE), under the nose (UN), center of the chin (CH), collarbone (CB), under the arm (UA), and the side of the hand or karate chop point (KC)[xxix].

How to do simple EFT (Tapping).

---

[6] The Skeptical Inquirer dismissed it as 'a hodgepodge of concepts derived from a variety of sources, primarily the ancient Chinese concept of *chi* (life-force)'

1) **Identify the issue**. The first thing to do is to identify the issue that is troubling you. It doesn't have to be complicated, you might just say, 'afraid of a bad diagnosis', 'worry about son travelling overseas', 'scared of going in a plane in case it crashes'---whatever is troubling you at the time.

2) **Test the intensity of the issue**. Rank the issue on a scale of 1-10, with 10 the most distressing. If you are not currently experiencing the issue, then imagine it as best you can. You use this to work out if the tapping technique has been effective.

Setup phrase. Start each round of tapping by saying a simple phrase and say it continuously while tapping the KC point. By doing this you acknowledge the problem, and accept yourself. The phrase is, **"even though I have this *ISSUE*, I deeply and completely accept myself"**. Using one of the examples above, I might say, 'even though I am terrified of cancer, I deeply and completely accept myself'[7].

You can be flexible with this, as not all issues fit into this; you could say, 'even though I am afraid of flying...' or 'even though my knee is sore...' Also, it is important to identify YOUR issue, and not someone else's (if it is someone else's issue, you could say, 'even though I feel really worried about my son traveling overseas...'). Note too, it's important to focus on the NEGATIVE. As with RAIN, it acknowledges and recognises emotions instead of burying them.

3) **The EFT sequence**[xxx]. You do not need to say the whole phrase as you tap, you just say part of it such as 'terrified of cancer' or 'worried about my son'. Then tap each of the points 3 to 10 times in the following sequence, WHILST saying the phrase aloud or to yourself if you are in a public place (i.e. an aeroplane):
   a. Top of the head (TOH)
   b. Beginning of the eyebrow (EB)

---

[7] Note, even just writing this makes me feel anxious...maybe I should do a couple of rounds of tapping!

c. Side of the eye (SE)
   d. Under the eye (UE)
   e. Under the nose (UN)
   f. Chin point (CH)
   g. Beginning of the collarbone (CB), and
   h. Under the arm (UA).

4) **5. Re-assess the intensity.** Now, assess your issue from 1-10 in terms of how much it is distressing you. Keep doing the tapping until the intensity goes below about 5.

You can tap as many times as you think necessary, and repeat the sequence as many times as you like until the problem seems not as insurmountable. People might look at you funny if you do it in public, but you can do it privately (I sometimes do it in my car). I'm not sure how tapping works, but it is really effective in the thick of an intense emotion.

Anxiety Forums

I include this in crisis techniques, because I only look at anxiety forums when I am going through a crisis. This is NOT the same as 'Googling' (**NEVER EVER GOOGLE!**) There are hundreds of anxiety forums on the internet, though only a few that are regularly updated and have a large community who are willing to help those who post the forums. I tend to avoid Facebook Groups, as they are not anonymous and often people can be quite hurtful, but obviously, if you like FB Groups, there are lots out there.

So, why are anxiety forums so useful? First, reading about other people's anxiety issues is a great way to 'ground' yourself and put your problems into perspective. Very often, you will read the story of someone who HAS been diagnosed with your specific dread disease---and is still alive and dealing with it. I find stories of people who have had cancer (often more than one type, and more than once) go a long way to easing some of my own fears. Like any support group, hearing other people tell their stories is a great way for you to feel that you are not abnormal, and that there are other people who have the same or similar problems.

Secondly, you can ask for advice on the forums. They can provide a (mostly) supportive forum for asking questions about what you are worried about, and reading other people's similar issues. You can post a question about what you are worried about, and there will inevitably be someone who has had an almost identical problem that turned out to be nothing serious, or if serious, found it and was cured (ignore the minority who tell anecdotes about their friend or family members with negative endings)! People on these forums all (mostly) have health anxiety, and respect your boundaries. Think what you may of trigger words etc. but most participants are careful with words (i.e. they talk about C instead of cancer). Forums are also great for discussions about different therapies, medication, possible side effects etc.

With forums, please update the thread if you have had a problem and it has turned out to be benign/ nothing serious/ etc. This really helps others searching for similar issues (or sets of symptoms).

Thirdly, the majority of forums are not just discussion boards, often they have a huge collection of resources, articles, blogs, wikis and pinned/recommended posts. These can be enormously helpful.

Finally, sometimes in forums, you get someone who is so obsessed about a tiny insignificant symptom (often with multiple photos attached) that other forum members start to get annoyed with them. While people on anxiety forums are often extremely supportive, if a person posts repeatedly about something, that has been investigated and tested by multiple medical specialists, and they *still* don't believe them, then even they get irritated!

Many people (if not everyone) have a tendency to be hard on themselves, what Buddhists call the second arrow. By this, they mean, that you do the behavior (the first arrow, which hurts you), then you chastise yourself for the behavior (by say, calling yourself an idiot), thus hurt yourself again with the second arrow. This is very counter-intuitive (and would probably appall Buddhist practitioners) but I use the second arrow tendency to 'kick myself out' of anxiety states, imagining that others think I am annoying and persistent. I don't necessarily recommend you do this to yourself, but it often works to snap **me** out of an anxiety episode.

Some useful anxiety forums (that in some cases, are sub forums of larger ones---don't go up to the actual medical conditions ones, unless you are feeling masochistic) are:

- **Health Anxiety (part of Anxiety Central)**[xxxi]. Anxiety Central has a large collection of resources. I cannot find who owns or runs this site, but it is very useful, and is updated regularly. It seems to be based in the USA
- **Health Boards Anxiety Message Board**[xxxii]. This one is part of a larger healthboards forum on just about any medical topic (avoid some of these if they are your trigger fears). This US based site has a lot of useful information although the anxiety sub-board is less regularly used than some others, and does not have a specific section on health anxiety.
- **Health Anxiety: No More Panic**[xxxiii]. This UK based site is extremely rich in information, and if you post on it, you will almost always get a reply relatively quickly. You can also search by topic, and it will bring up other posts that are on a similar topic. It has lots of 'sticky' posts, and on the main page, heaps of resources on various types of anxiety. This site is particularly useful.

Best Friend technique

Commonly, anxious people are embarrassed about their fears. This is partly due to societal attitudes about mental health and partly due to the Buddhist concept of the 'second arrow' where you beat yourself up about a feeling or something you have done (thus hurting yourself twice). Often, someone will suffer agonies of anxiety whilst at the same time as pretending to everyone else that all is fine (most people who know you very well will pick up on this however, but if you are relatively introverted, you may not have a wide group of friends or close family to support you). Sometimes too, people will mock you or make fun of your anxiety or tell you to 'just think positively'!

When this is the case, there is the 'best friend technique'[xxxiv]. A real best friend works well but you can also use an imaginary best friend or therapist. There's a couple of ways you can do this, and the first is to imagine your friend or therapist in the same position, confiding in you. So, say your friend comes up to you and says, I am really struggling now, because I am really anxious about X symptom or feeling. Then, imagine that you are giving advice to your best friend. You may gently tell him or her that they are being unrealistic, but you are not going to be mean or mock them. How would you advise your best friend if they had the same problem?

Another way you can do this is to imagine that the things you tell yourself, you are telling your best friend. We often tell ourselves, without even being aware of doing this, terrible things, like 'I am stupid', 'I am an idiot, how can I think that way', 'nobody will ever love me if I am so stressed out and anxious', and a trillion other ways that we put ourselves down. Now, imagine saying the same things to someone you love. Would you tell your best friend that they are stupid, or that nobody will ever love them? Of course not! Well, if you do, you probably don't have any best friends!

What is the benefit of NOT finding out

I can't remember where I read this, I seem to recall it was regarding something totally different than health anxiety. This is one of those tips and tricks that work when you are in a doctor avoiding situation (rather than the opposite). For example, you are overdue for a regular test, or the government (as in Australia) sends you a letter that your mammogram is due or you receive your annual bowel cancer detection kit in the mail, and you are too terrified to go for the test *in case they find something!*

Using this technique, you ask yourself, 'what is the **benefit** of **NOT** finding out?' So, if you are terrified of a certain disease, and you get a symptom which *may* indicate that disease, and you ignore it, what is the benefit? Obviously, if it turns out to be a type of cancer or heart disease, and you ignore it, there are only DISbenefits to not finding out. This is a bit counter-intuitive to people with health anxiety, as they are either going to the doctor every week, or avoiding them entirely. But if you ask yourself, how will I benefit by ignoring the symptom (i.e. what if they do find something), then you may just realise that finding something early is way better than leaving it too late.

Dumb ways to die

I'm not sure if this is an actual way of helping with health anxiety but it works for me. In the last episode that I had, I was obsessed with skin cancer (and an incredibly rare and aggressive form, and for which I had zero risk factors---who said health anxiety was rational); so I started thinking, what *other* ways are there to die than what I was afraid of?

So, what I did was think of the hundreds and thousands of ways that I could die, and as I walked my dog, I would list them, in categories (because I am rather OCD as well as anxious).

Now you might think that for a person with health anxiety to list ways to die would be really stressful; but most of us with health anxiety have a specific disease or group of disease about which they are anxious. So, if I am afraid of certain cancers for instance, I am not particularly afraid of heart disease (which is somewhat silly as most of my grandparents died of various cardiovascular disease related causes and none of them from cancer.

Anyway, so I started with listing non-illness related causes of death; and to make this a little less stressful, really odd and unlikely ones, like being hit by a meteorite, or like the story I heard of someone's relative who was terrified of flying, but refused to take the train, because---*an aeroplane might crash on it*!

Then I started listing unlikely death from diseases that I had zero chance of getting, like kuru which is a prion based disease you get from eating the brains of your dead relatives. Given that I have no desire whatsoever to eat the brains of anyone, relatives or not, even if I am in an air crash in the Andes, I figure I'm pretty safe from kuru.

Like the above, the benefit of not finding out, it seems a bit counterintuitive but it works really well (at least for me). It may also work quite well because of some of the other techniques listed, such as progressive densensitisation which is used in phobia therapy. If you think of various ways that you could die, then you are facing the concept of death...your death. Perhaps by listing extremely weird ways to die helps you acknowledge your mortality.

A similar way I do this is to think about the diseases I fear the most, and think, yes, well, that spot could be cancer, but at least you can see it, if it changes, and then get it checked out. You can't see inside things, and some have no symptoms at all! This won't work if you are deathly afraid of symptomless diseases, but it may help with desensitisation.

CONCLUSION

This is not one of those self-help books that promise THE cure for your disease, THE definitive guide to weight loss, making friends, becoming a millionaire, etc. People buy those all the time, but they are just full of empty promises. There are no magic bullets, and if it sounds too good to be true, then it probably is. I would love to say that I have THE cure for health anxiety (I'd definitely use it on myself first) but I don't. However, I hope the information, techniques and resources in this book can help you.

We are all different, and all of our anxieties, whatever the label, are different. They also have different causes, symptoms and duration. Because of this, a technique might work brilliantly for one person, and be a total dud for the next. This book is a list of techniques that I have found useful, and that others have found useful.

"Since death will take us anyway, why live our life in fear? Why not die in our old ways and be free to live?" Jack Kornfield

STORIES OF HEALTH ANXIETY

THINGS I HAVE THOUGHT I WAS DYING FROM (AND THE REAL CAUSE)

Symptom	My Diagnosis	Real Cause
Bitten by rat	Rabies	Anxiety from rat bite
Bitten by dog	Rabies	Dog bite (dog still alive)
Pins & needles & dizziness	Snake bite (nonexistent)	Hyperventilation & anxiety
Palpitations	Heart attack	Anxiety
Palpitations	Heart attack	Panic attack
Palpitations	Heart attack	PAC (still might kill me!)
Horrible black spot	Merkel Cell Carcinoma	Infected splinter
White mark on foot	Melanoma	Scar
Horrible looking mole	Melanoma	Freckle
Lump on thigh	Sarcoma	Lipoma
Red pee	Cancer	Beetroot
Yellow pee	Cancer	Berocca
Smelly pee	Cancer	Asparagus
Red poo	Cancer	Too much beetroot
Red poo	Cancer	Fell on bum & cut skin
Vaginal bleeding	Cancer	(very infrequent) post-menopausal sex & no lube
Sore ribs & back	Liver cancer	Bad posture & anxiety
Sore jaw	Tetanus	Grinding teeth from anxiety
Sore jaw	Cancer	Tooth infection
Swollen lymph glands	Cancer	Tooth infection
Lump on arm	Nodular melanoma	Pimple
Lump in boob	Cancer	Fibroadenoma
Back pain	Cancer	Bad posture & anxiety (but the jury is still out lol)

Back pain	Cancer	Lifting a piano!
Back pain	Cancer	Hiking 300km over the Alps and not training
Back pain	Cancer	Falling & twisting back
Chin hairs not growing fast	Something fatal no doubt	Age
Nails with ridges	Something fatal no doubt	Age
Black rings under eyes	Something fatal no doubt	Sleeping with cats
Nasty black spot	Kaposi's Sarcoma	Cigarette burn
Lump under arm	Cancer	Infected hair follicle
Headache	Cancer	Flu/ Sinus
Headache	Cancer	Red wine
Stomach problems	Cancer	Gas
Stomach problems	Cancer	Zoloft
Wheezing	Asthma	Crying whilst running a marathon (was tired)
Couldn't breathe properly in night	Lung cancer	Panic attack
Diarrhea	Cancer	Anxiety/ Zoloft
Frequent bruising	Cancer	Being clumsy

A PERSONAL STORY OF HEALTH ANXIETY

I discovered <horrors> a hard lump on my ankle, just inside my right ankle bone. Surprisingly for me, I didn't worry much at first, as I had bashed that exact spot with a garden mattock about a month ago, then had re-hurt it twice more, resulting in a horrible bruise. As I have said before, I am horrendously clumsy. Anyway, I did poke and prod at it, but figured it was from the mattock whacking episode.

However, after a few weeks, it didn't go away, so I started poking and prodding in earnest. I would lift my foot up on to my bathroom sink and turn on the makeup mirror and peer myopically at my ankle (luckily I am flexible) and feel the dimensions of the lump. Was it getting any bigger, was it changing, was it going away?

One day, I noticed that it was sort of sticking out, and had what looked like a tiny vein on the top of it. A hard lump…with a vein! My brain went into instant cancer fear mode! That *must* mean it was a tumour! OMG, I was going to die! I started poking and prodding in earnest, and not only did it start changing colour, it began to hurt too.

Now it was a nasty sticky out looking thing, which hurt, and which was purply red, like a blood blister, but not really soft. Sometimes I persuaded myself that it was squishy, and thus some sort of cyst, but other times, it seemed really hard. It also seemed better in the mornings and swelled up in the evenings. (Almost certainly due to the lack of poking and prodding and squeezing whilst slumbering).

I finally gave in and consulted Dr Google, who reassured me, that with the exception of melanoma, cancers of the feet and ankle were exceptionally rare. Phew! I relaxed for about 2 days, until I read a cartoon on Facebook (yes, a cartoon…on Facebook!) about someone who had sarcoma of the foot!

I instantly panicked and made a doctor's appointment. The doctor peered at the lump with an illuminated magnifying glass (what I know as the skin cancer inspection device) then prodded at it, and asked me if I had injured it. Yes, I said, and told him what I had done. He said, stop poking and prodding at it, you are making it worse. It is just scar tissue and blood clotting, and should go away in about 6 weeks. I didn't tell him that I had hurt it more than 6 weeks ago.

I relaxed, for at least a day, until I Googled sarcoma; nope, that wasn't it. I half thought it was nodular melanoma, but it had, after all, started UNDER the skin and not on it. So I put a Band-Aid on it and left it alone (well, more or less alone, I would lift up the flap of the Band-Aid every couple of days and hurriedly peer at it to reassure myself that it wasn't growing any bigger). It didn't look any bigger, but it was still red and purple and horrible looking.

Now, this whole time, I was wearing long socks, in case, you know, someone would actually see the horrible lesion and say, oh my goodness me, you should get that looked at! I avoided going to places where I had to expose the ghastly thing, such as yoga and the swimming pool and the beach, and I bathed every night by candlelight, not for romantic reasons, but so as not to have to see the tumorous ankle. I may add, by the way, that although the lump looked awful, it was actually quite small, around 2mm, and no-one would have noticed. I also started looking obsessively at people's ankles, to see if anyone else had something similar. They must have thought that I was a bit odd.

After about two weeks, I took the Band-Aid off, and left it off overnight. The next morning, it was no better, in fact it looked worse. I started Googling in earnest, until on about page 900 of a site of skin disorders, I found a horrible looking picture that looked just like the awful ankle tumor! It was a type of very rare and highly aggressive skin cancer called Merkel Cell Carcinoma! Oh my god! That must be it! And it was bound to have metastasized already. My catastrophizing went into overdrive. What music would they play at my funeral? Must I change my will? Where would I find a nice hospice?

I ignored the fact that this was an exceptionally rare type of cancer, grew very fast (mine hadn't grown at all), and mostly affected men over 70 with fair skin on the head and torso and with depressed immune systems (none of which, of course, applied to me). By the way, don't Google pictures of that disease if you have a sensitive stomach.

Now in full anxiety mode, I made another appointment with another doctor, supposedly for my annual PAP smear for cervical cancer, which I am, surprisingly not in the least afraid, which is completely idiotic, as I have a far higher chance of getting that, given my extremely misspent youth. After all the stuff, I produced the lesion and asked the doctor about it. She looked at it, asked if I had injured it, and said, oh that is just scar tissue and blood clotting. Leave it alone, and it should go away...in about 6 months!

Slightly reassured as it had only been there for 3 months, and hadn't grown, I reapplied the Band-Aid, and left it sort of alone. After about 3 weeks however, it was still the same, but now was definitely quite squishy. I decided that instead of Merkel Cell Carcinoma, it was nodular melanoma, so I started poking and prodding at my groin in case I had swollen glands!

A week later, I took off the Band-Aid after my bath, and it was sticking up and very squishy, so I thought, stuff it, and got a needle, some Dettol and some matches. I had previously resisted the urge to self-operate because I figured that if it was cancerous, the act of sticking a needle in it would be bound to release cancer cells and I would die sooner. Obviously, although I am hypochondriac and thus have a superb knowledge of potentially fatal diseases, I am not really an expert on tumours.

So, I stuck the needle into it and squeezed. Out came blood and pus! Lots of blood and pus! It was a bloody (lol) abscess! Then, something stuck out. Oh my god, maybe it was a bit of bone, and it was bone cancer, and my ankle bone was fragmenting. I pulled it out and peered at it. It was a SPLINTER of wood! I had had a splinter in my ankle for nearly 4 months! No wonder it had hurt and not wanted to heal. The Band-Aid had probably drawn it out!

Funny enough, after that, it got better, and the lump went away though now I do actually have a tiny black spot left over, which IS blood clotting and scar tissue!

REFERENCES

[i] Western Australia Centre for Clinical Interventions (CCI). 2016. https://www.cci.health.wa.gov.au/Resources/Looking-After-Yourself/Health-Anxiety

[i] Black Dog Institute, 2016, What is Anxiety? https://www.blackdoginstitute.org.au/clinical-resources/anxiety/what-is-anxiety

[ii] CCI. http://www.cci.health.wa.gov.au/resources/infopax.cfm?Info_ID=53

[i] Beyond Blue. Statistics and References. https://www.beyondblue.org.au/about-us/research-projects/statistics-and-references

[ii] Leon F Seltzer, Evolution of the Self. Trauma and the Freeze Response: Good, Bad, or Both? https://www.psychologytoday.com/blog/evolution-the-self/201507/trauma-and-the-freeze-response-good-bad-or-both

[iii] Dubuc, Bruno, The evolutionary lives of the brain, http://thebrain.mcgill.ca/flash/d/d_05/d_05_cr/d_05_cr_her/d_05_cr_her.html

[iv] Tara Brach. 2017. Radical Self Honesty. The joy of getting real. https://www.tarabrach.com/radical-self-honesty-joy/

[v] Tara Brach. 2017. Radical Self Honesty. The joy of getting real. https://www.tarabrach.com/radical-self-honesty-joy/

[vi] Anxiety - symptoms, treatment and causes, Mind Health Connect. https://www.mindhealthconnect.org.au/anxiety

[vii] Beyond Blue. Types of Anxiety. https://www.beyondblue.org.au/the-facts/anxiety/types-of-anxiety

[viii] Black Dog Institute, 2016. What is anxiety. https://www.blackdoginstitute.org.au/clinical-resources/anxiety/what-is-anxiety

[ix] Abraham, M. 2018. A Brief History of Anxiety. https://www.calmclinic.com/brief-history-of-anxiety

[x] Torres, L. 2017. The 4 Main Criticisms Of The DSM-5. https://www.theodysseyonline.com/criticisms-dsm-5

[xi] NHS Website, no date, What is Health Anxiety? http://www.nhs.uk/conditions/hypochondria/Pages/Introduction.aspx

[xii] Source: Centre for Clinical Interventions, WA Health Service, 2011 Helping health anxiety. Module 1, Understanding Health Anxiety, p.4; http://www.cci.health.wa.gov.au/resources/infopax.cfm?Info_ID=53?

[xiii] WebMD, no date, Somatic Symptom and Related Disorders, http://www.webmd.com/mental-health/somatoform-disorders-symptoms-

types-treatment
xiv Harvard Medical School, 2017. Anxiety and physical illness. Understanding and treating anxiety can often improve the outcome of chronic disease. https://www.health.harvard.edu/staying-healthy/anxiety_and_physical_illness
xv Cancer Council of Australia. Position Statement on Alcohol. https://wiki.cancer.org.au/policy/Position_statement_-_Alcohol_and_cancer
i McGregor, N. 2015. Seven new genes linked to anxiety disorders https://theconversation.com/seven-new-genes-linked-to-anxiety-disorders-42835
ii Norrholm, S & Ressler, K.J. 2009. Genetics of Anxiety and Trauma-Related Disorders https://www.ncbi.nlm.nih.gov/pmc/articles/PMC2760665/
iii The Guardian, 2014. Epigenetics 101: a beginner's guide to explaining everything. https://www.theguardian.com/science/occams-corner/2014/apr/25/epigenetics-beginners-guide-to-everything
iv Kirkpatrick, B. 2016. Inherited Epigenetic and Behavioral Consequences of Trauma Could be Reversed. https://www.whatisepigenetics.com/inherited-epigenetic-and-behavioral-consequences-of-trauma-could-be-reversed/
v What is epigenetics. DNA methylation. ND. https://www.whatisepigenetics.com/dna-methylation/
vi Gregoire, C. 2015. The Surprising Link Between Gut Bacteria And Anxiety. http://www.huffingtonpost.com.au/entry/gut-bacteria-mental-healt_n_6391014
vii BioMed Central. New light on link between gut bacteria and anxiety. ScienceDaily. 2017. https://www.sciencedaily.com/releases/2017/08/170824221455.htm
viii Insurance Journal, 2015. Worried About Dying from Surgery, Hurricane, Plane Crash? Check Out the Odds. http://www.insurancejournal.com/news/national/2015/06/01/370141.htm
ix Business Insider, 2017. How likely are foreign terrorists to kill Americans? The odds may surprise you Read more at https://www.businessinsider.com/death-risk-statistics-terrorism-disease-accidents-2017-1#M3BaaaHxY7HL3MWX.99
x Zimbardo, P. 2009. The Psychology of Time. TED Talk transcript. https://www.ted.com/talks/philip_zimbardo_prescribes_a_healthy_take_on_time/transcript
xi Sword, R. 2011. Time Perspective Therapy. http://www.timeperspectivetherapy.org/time-perspectives/
xii Zimbardo, P. 2008. Time Perspective Biases: General, Phenomenological Characterizations of each Time Perspective. http://www.thetimeparadox.com/2008/08/03/an-overview-of-time-perspective-types

xiii Papastamatelou, J., Unger, A., Giotakos, O., & Athanasiadou, F. 2015. Is Time Perspective a Predictor of Anxiety and Perceived Stress? Some Preliminary Results from Greece.
https://link.springer.com/article/10.1007/s12646-015-0342-6
xiv If you are interested in pursuing this further, you can do the Zimbardo Time Perspectives Test yourself here (http://www.thetimeparadox.com/zimbardo-time-perspective-inventory/).
xv ABC. Scott, S. 2015. Australians cut back on or stopped taking statins following ABC Catalyst story, researchers find. http://www.abc.net.au/news/2015-06-15/patients-cut-back-on-statins-after-catalyst-story-research/6545026
xvi Healthline Australia. ND. Statins, the pros and cons.
https://www.healthline.com/health/high-cholesterol/statins-pros-cons#definition
xvii Collier, N.S. 2008. Avoiding the second arrow.
http://www.nscblog.com/miscellaneous/avoiding-the-second-arrow/
xviii Tara Brach. 2011. Learning to Respond not React.
http://blog.tarabrach.com/2011/08/learning-to-respond-not-react.html
i Rayner S. 2015. Why the Menopause Creates a Perfect Storm for Anxiety.
https://www.psychologytoday.com/blog/worry-and-panic/201503/why-the-menopause-creates-perfect-storm-anxiety
ii Cancer Council of Australia. ND. Known and Probable Human Carcinogens.
https://www.cancer.org/cancer/cancer-causes/general-info/known-and-probable-human-carcinogens.html
iii Shearer, H. 2017. Breaking the Booze Habit.
https://www.amazon.com/Breaking-Booze-Habit-Seinfelds-habitual/dp/1974342662
iv Wei, M. 2017. New Research Shows Depression Linked with Inflammation.
https://www.psychologytoday.com/au/blog/urban-survival/201701/new-research-shows-depression-linked-inflammation
i CCI Modules 3&6, WA Government
ii Dixon. 2017. Revolutionary blood test 'can predict how long you'll LIVE' (*not necessarily authoritative, given the source*). https://www.express.co.uk/life-style/health/750728/blood-test-how-long-people-live-life-span-science-death-ageing
iii James Randi Educational Foundation. ND. http://web.randi.org/home/jref-status
iv Anxiety Central Forum. ND. List of over 100 Anxiety Symptoms.

http://www.anxiety-central.com/topic/75-list-of-over-100-anxiety-symptoms/
i Gleisner, G. 2016. What is CBT?
https://www.psychologytoday.com/au/blog/bottoms/201611/what-is-cbt
ii Mayo Clinic. ND. Cognitive Behavioral Therapy.
https://www.mayoclinic.org/tests-procedures/cognitive-behavioral-

therapy/about/pac-20384610
iii American Psychological Association. ND. What is Exposure Therapy. Clinical Guideline. http://www.apa.org/ptsd-guideline/patients-and-families/exposure-therapy.aspx
iv Queensland Brain Institute. 2018. New pathway to extinguish fearful memories discovere. https://qbi.uq.edu.au/article/2018/04/new-pathway-extinguish-fearful-memories-discovered
v Mayo Clinic. 2004. Selective serotonin reuptake inhibitors (SSRIs). https://www.mayoclinic.org/diseases-conditions/depression/in-depth/ssris/art-20044825
vi Ooi S.L., Henderson P. & Pak S.C. 2018. Kava for Generalized Anxiety Disorder: A Review of Current Evidence. https://www.ncbi.nlm.nih.gov/pubmed/29641222
vii WebMD. ND. Kava. https://www.webmd.com/vitamins/ai/ingredientmono-872/kava
viii Sporteluxe. 2017. I Tried CBD Oil To Deal With Anxiety—Here's My Honest Review. https://sporteluxe.com/tried-cbd-oil-help-anxiety-heres-honest-review/
ix Villines, Z. 2018. Can CBD oil help anxiety? https://www.medicalnewstoday.com/articles/319622.php
x Therapeutic Goods Administration, Australian Government. 2018. Claims about hemp and CBD oils misleading consumers. https://www.tga.gov.au/behind-news/claims-about-hemp-and-cbd-oils-misleading-consumers
xi Greenberg, G. 2018. Claims about hemp and CBD oils misleading consumers. New York Times Magazine. https://www.nytimes.com/2018/11/07/magazine/placebo-effect-medicine.html
xii Moseley JB, O'Malley K, Petersen NJ, et al. A controlled trial of arthroscopic surgery for osteoarthritis of the knee. N Engl J Med. 2002 Jul 11;347(2):81–8. PubMed #12110735. https://www.painscience.com/biblio/fascinating-landmark-study-of-placebo-surgery-for-knee-osteoarthritis.html
xiii Ferris, R. 2016. Powerful hallucinogens reduce anxiety and depression in cancer patients. https://www.cnbc.com/2016/12/02/powerful-hallucinogens-reduce-anxiety-and-depression-in-cancer-patients.html
xiv Wikipedia. ND. Meditation. https://en.wikipedia.org/wiki/Meditation
xv Tara Brach. 2013. (adapted from). True Refuge: Finding Peace & Freedom in Your Own Awakened Heart. Bantam. https://www.tarabrach.com/articles-interviews/rain-workingwithdifficulties/
xvi Ingraham, P. 2018. When to Worry About Low Back Pain And when not to! What's bark and what's bite? https://www.painscience.com/articles/when-to-worry-about-low-back-pain-and-when-not-to.php
xvii Death Café Australia website. http://deathcafe.com/c/Australia/

[xviii] Death Café international website. http://deathcafe.com/what/
[xix] Tara Brach website. https://www.tarabrach.com/
[xx] Byron Katie website. http://thework.com/en
[xxi] The Anxiety Guy Podcast. https://itunes.apple.com/gb/podcast/the-anxiety-guy-podcast/id1080900600?mt=2
[xxii] Novotny, S. & Kravitz, L. ND. The Science of Breathing https://www.unm.edu/~lkravitz/Article%20folder/Breathing.html
[xxiii] Wim Hof. ND. What is the Wim Hof Method? http://www.icemanwimhof.com/wim-hof-exercises
[xxiv] Boorman, J. ND. Wim Hof Method Explained & Benefits of Cold Exposure. http://placeofpersistence.com/wim-hof-method-explained-benefits-of-cold-exposure/
[xxv] CCI. https://www.cci.health.wa.gov.au/Resources/Looking-After-Yourself/Health-Anxiety
[xxvi] Tara Brach website. https://www.tarabrach.com/
[xxvii] Wells, S., Polglase, K., Andrews, H.B., Carrington, P. and Baker, A.H., 2003. Evaluation of a meridian-based intervention, Emotional Freedom Techniques (EFT), for reducing specific phobias of small animals. Journal of Clinical Psychology, 59(9), pp.943-966. http://www.eftdownunder.com/research-paper-evaluation-of-eft-for-reducing-specific-phobias/
[xxviii] Spencer-Rowland, M. 2017. What is EFT and how do you do it? https://livingnow.com.au/what-is-eft-and-how-do-you-do-it/
[xxix] Gary Craig. ND. How to do the EFT Tapping Basics - The Basic Recipe. https://www.emofree.com/nl/eft-tutorial/tapping-basics/how-to-do-eft.html
[xxx] Gary Craig. ND. EFT: Test driving the Basic Recipe by Founder Gary Craig. https://www.youtube.com/watch?v=kbBNaqsKatM
[xxxi] Anxiety Central. Health Anxiety Forum. http://www.anxiety-central.com/forum/9-health-anxiety/
[xxxiixxxii] Healthboards. Anxiety Forum. https://www.healthboards.com/boards/anxiety/
[xxxiii] No More Panic. Health Anxiety Forum. http://www.nomorepanic.co.uk/forumdisplay.php?f=29
[xxxiv] CBT Los Angeles. ND. Would You Really Tell THAT to a Friend? http://cogbtherapy.com/cbt-blog/2013/07/would-you-really-tell-that-to-friend.html

www.ingramcontent.com/pod-product-compliance
Lightning Source LLC
Chambersburg PA
CBHW030714220526
45463CB00005B/2044